THE SEVEN SACRED RITES OF MENOPAUSE

THE SPIRITUAL JOURNEY TO THE WISE-WOMAN YEARS

BY

KRISTI MEISENBACH BOYLAN

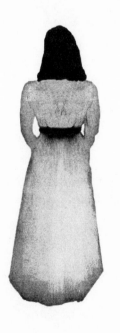

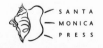

SANTA MONICA PRESS

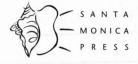

SANTA
MONICA
PRESS

Published by:
SANTA MONICA PRESS LLC
P.O. Box 1076
Santa Monica, CA 90406-1076
1-800-784-9553
www.santamonicapress.com

Printed in the United States

Santa Monica Press books are available at special quantity discounts when purchased in bulk by corporations, organizations, or groups. Please call our special sales department at 1-800-784-9553.

This book is intended to provide general information. The publisher, author, distributor, and copyright owner are not engaged in rendering health, medical, psychological, legal, financial, or other professional advice or services, and are not liable or responsible to any person or group with respect to any loss, illness, or injury caused or alleged to be caused by the information found in this book.

ISBN 1-891661-13-2

Library of Congress Cataloging-in-Publication Data

Meisenbach Boylan, Kristi, 1960-
    The seven sacred rites of menopause: the spiritual journey to the wise-woman years / by Kristi Meisenbach Boylan.
        p. cm.
    ISBN 1-891661-13-2
        1. Menopause—Popular works. 2. Menopause—
Psychological aspects—Popular works.
        I. Title.

RG186 .M426 2000
618.1'75—dc21   00-044542

Book cover design by Susan Landesmann
Book interior design by cooldogdesign

CONTENTS

APPENDIX

For my mother

and

my grandmothers

and

their grandmothers

and

theirs . . .

"Let the Circle Be Unbroken."

ACKNOWLEDGMENTS

MANY WOMEN, SEVERAL MEN and two children gave of their hearts and time so that this book could be published.

The women are almost too numerous to name, but I will give it a try. Many thanks to: Jo Harris, who was the first to share her journey and who, in fact, became the barge back for me; Mimi Meisenbach, Donna Phillips and Jody Neice, who held tightly to my hands during the darkest parts of the mist; all the women, including my grandmother, aunts and cousins, who bore witness to my menopausal journey and, in turn, allowed me to witness theirs; Claudette Bellocchio, who first told me the story of the Goddess; and most importantly, my mother,

Ann Meisenbach, who is herself the embodiment of the wise-woman-crone.

The several men who have been a part of my journey include, but are not limited to: Dr. John Woodward and Bob Scarbrough, who were relentless in finding the right dose of hormones for my system; my brothers, Kurt and Karl Meisenbach, who, although they never quite understood the journey, bore witness to it in their own loving ways; my father, David Meisenbach, who literally shares my dreams; and my husband, Patrick Boylan, whose love and loyalty to me over the last 15 years has astounded even the angels.

Although it is thought that children rarely comprehend the lives of their parents, I have been blessed with two very intuitive beings, who not only understood the journey, but inspired it. Thank you, Amanda and Brandan, for choosing me.

Last but not least, I must not forget all the people who took care of the business end of editing and publishing the Sacred Rites. To Jeffrey Goldman, and all his staff at Santa Monica Press who worked on this book, thank you for recognizing the importance of sharing the menopausal voyage.

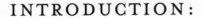

INTRODUCTION:
THE VOYAGE THROUGH MENOPAUSE

MY FIRST THOUGHTS were that I was going crazy. I was sure of it. I remember tearfully asking a close friend and neighbor if she would look out for my children in the event that I had a total nervous breakdown. After all, what else could possibly be causing the sudden and unexpected onset of memory lapses, anxiety, depression, night sweats, and phobia attacks that had completely turned my life upside down?

My initial visits with my internist had turned up nothing, further convincing me that I was losing my mind. Knowing that I was under a great deal of stress, this internist wrote me a prescription for

Klonopin and referred me to a psychiatrist. Thankfully, a friend intervened and reminded me of her own difficult passage through menopause. And since my mother had been attributing my nervousness to hormones, I agreed to see the endocrinologist that my friend had recommended. Still, I was sure that at 36 I was much too young to be going through the change. Much to my surprise, however, both my estrogen and progesterone levels came back extremely low—I was in menopause.

Angered by my internist's misdiagnosis of panic disorder, I armed myself with every manual I could find on this mysterious mid-life passage, and there were plenty. On the shelves of every library and bookstore were a dozen or so books with the word menopause in their title. The anatomical texts, most of which were written by well-meaning health care professionals, offered advice on lessening the physical and emotional ailments that accompany the inevitable hormonal decline. Whether to take hormone replacement therapy (HRT) or to "tough it out naturally" seemed to be the question of the day for transitioning women.

Although the advice and expertise of the healing community was certainly educational (more than 50 million women will be going through menopause in the year 2005), the information still wasn't enough to satisfy my need to understand what was happening to me. I kept reading and searching, wanting to find out more. Yes, I knew what it meant to be in perimenopause. I knew that estrogen loss increased the risk of osteoporosis and heart disease. I knew also, from personal experience, that it brought on mood swings and a whole host of other emotional and physical problems. But what else was going on? What was really happening to me?

Even as I asked myself that question, I sensed, as every woman does, that menopause wasn't just about the cessation of a monthly cycle. And it wasn't about getting old and dry and wrinkly, either. Deep within me I knew that this experience called menopause would somehow turn into a voyage, a journey, a time-consuming pilgrimage that might take years to complete. And it would be a journey that would not only transform my body, but would transform my soul as well.

And so while my endocrinologist began the arduous task of balancing my hormone levels, I, armed with a gut feeling and a large dose of uncertainty, began the arduous task of uncovering what the spiritual journey of menopause encompassed.

I started with the written word. But nothing connecting spirituality with menopause could be found in the two dozen or so books I had faithfully purchased from my local bookstore. In fact, there wasn't even a short listing in any of the indexes on spirit. I was disappointed but not discouraged. After all, most of the books on menopause were written by medical doctors and physicians were trained to heal the body, not the soul.

My next step was to go straight to the source. I talked with my mother, my grandmother, my aunts, and every other woman over 50 who would tolerate my intrusive questioning. My search eventually led me to internet chat rooms, where, not so surprisingly, I found the reassurance and answers I had been looking for.

These women were not the least bit shy about sharing their spiritual transformation with me. Not only did I receive an enormous amount of information on what to expect over the next few years, I learned a lot about the chutzpah of post-menopausal women who are allowed to share their experiences over the internet without the fear of someone shaming them. And as I corresponded with these women, I also began to document my own journey through menopause. As I did, I learned a few truths about the menopausal spirit.

One of the most enduring lessons I learned was that the menopausal life passage isn't about a woman's body fighting to right itself of hormone imbalances at all. It is really about the soul trying to right itself of spiritual imbalances; it is about a woman's spirit fighting to regain a sense of symmetry in a distorted, asymmetrical world.

Though unbalanced hormones are certainly a symptom of the passage, it is the heart's cry to once again be absolute, and the spirit's desire to return to the place where it can exist in its natural state of strength and courage that defines the real journey through menopause.

And I learned that the menopausal pilgrimage was about returning to that place, that sacred land at the core of the soul, called home. And in returning to that home, that inner sanctum, a woman would again find that sense of spiritual strength and wholeness that she craved, and she would once again be filled with the zest and self-reliance that she had before puberty and children and her husband lured her away.

In addition to enlightening me about the spiritual truths behind menopause, these women also gave me a lot of down-to-earth advice about the myths and fallacies that surround the physical transformation.

One of the most widespread misconceptions I discovered was that menopause was an event that happens to a woman around the age of 51. Although the average age of completing menopause may be 51, many women begin experiencing symptoms as early as 35. This means that menopause can often take up to ten or more years. And so the process of birthing oneself, which is what a woman does as she moves through menopause, becomes a lengthy one indeed.

An obstetrician was once asked how long it takes for a child to be born. He answered "it takes as long as it takes." And so it is with menopause. It takes as long as it takes. The menopausal quest to retrieve that sense of wholeness is a pilgrimage that cannot be rushed, and it is important for a woman (and her loved ones) to keep in mind that one doesn't travel to the inner sanctum of the female soul and back overnight.

For the very reason that menopause is such a lengthy transition and not just a threshold, I feel that the journey should not be classified as a solitary rite of passage, but rather as a succession of rites or rituals. These succession of rites mark a woman's way through mid-life, validating the pain and frustration of her voyage like stepping stones across a rising river. Robert Fulghum wrote in his book *From Beginning to End: The Rituals of Our Lives* that "rituals are one way in which attention is paid." I have found this to be true for the rituals of menopause. The stepping stones of rites from childbearer to crone draw a woman's attention to her changing body, and more importantly, they draw attention to her changing spirit.

In chronicling my own lengthy voyage and those of my postmenopausal friends, I have discovered that there are seven distinct rituals, or rites, that a woman may expect to participate in during her menopausal journey. I believe that these rites and the accompanying feelings that occur with them should not be looked at as isolated stages, though. Instead, they should be viewed as a string of connecting rituals that, in some form or another, have been performed by millions of women for, perhaps, millions of years.

Furthermore, I believe that the seven ceremonial milestones that a woman encounters along the way should be viewed as celebrations, not as symptoms of illness or disease. And they should not be treated as silent acts, either. The rites are commemorations of our womanhood, and should be shared and talked about. Like all female rituals, such as childbirth or monthly cramps, the menopausal rites are not meant as a punishment from God or nature, but are a way of waking us up to being truly female. They are part of the invaluable lessons bestowed upon us by our Creator that, from the very beginning, set us apart from men. These sacred rites are also a road map, a sort of diagram to chart our course—a way of understanding where we've been and where we are headed. And more importantly, they are a reminder of just how long we stayed away, and just how far we've come in finding our way back home.

I would also like to add that although the information I gathered did seem to repeat itself in many places, it was still apparent that this unity of sisterhood wasn't exactly the same for all women. I have found that as each woman makes her way through these rites, she will find herself on an unprecedented, uncharted course. Some may find the sacraments painful, while others may hardly notice them. The journey of menopause is a highly individualistic passage, for even as all women make the voyage, the currents each chooses to sail on are hers and hers alone.

As I gathered my information and put these truths together, I knew that it was important for me to relate what I had found to other women, who, like me, were searching for a deeper meaning to the transition of menopause. I wanted to present the information in a way that would be meaningful as well as entertaining, and most importantly, I wanted the rites to resonate with the archetypical places that lie deep in the core of the female soul. One of the most renowned sites that came to mind was the land of Camelot.

Like many women, I treasure the legends of King Arthur, not because of the chivalry or stories of love and romance, but because of the tales of Avalon. Avalon, that mystical, magical island that floated in the mists was where "real" women lived. It was a land where women ruled as priestesses and God had a feminine face. It was a place where women were truly whole.

And so, in this book, I have chosen to use that mythical island of Avalon as a point of reference to describe the place where menopausal women go to recover their wholeness. For this purpose, Avalon will represent the sacred island that lies within the mists of a woman's soul where she can go and retrieve the part of herself that was left behind during her childbearing years.

This sacred voyage isn't just about travelling to Avalon, though. It's also about bringing back a piece of the island forever planted in one's heart. It's about retrieving that inner sanctum where women are free to draw down the moon or share their gift of sight without fear of being burned at the stake, and bringing it back to the outer world where intuition still falls under the category of occult. In fact, a vital part of the menopausal healing process can only be completed by reclaiming that ancient golden elixir of the crone and bringing back the wisdom from it to share with the rest of the planet. So while this pilgrimage of menopause is about journeying within, it's also a pilgrimage of journeying out as well.

Although this book is a spiritual guide and not intended to be a substitute for medical care during the menopausal years, I have included some basic information on the female anatomy, along with some helpful hints on making the transition easier. I hope you find the information helpful, and I wish you all the best on your own voyage into the wise-woman years.

THE FIRST RITE:

SUMMONING THE BARGE

DEEP WITHIN THE hidden layers of our very being is a mechanism that holds time, an alarm clock for the soul that activates the body as well. Or maybe it is actually an alarm for the body that calls out to the soul. Either way, as all things in the body and soul are intertwined, this unique apparatus has a direct connection to Great Grandfather Time.

This unseen mechanism is what calls us from our mother's womb, beckoning us into the world. It is the same mechanism that as babies prompts us into the toddler stage by urging us to walk. In fact, it is the timekeeper of every stage of our life, right into puberty and on into death, when again, it calls on the body to shut down. It is this same timekeeper that also determines the exact moment for a woman to begin her voyage into menopause, and it is what summons the vessel to take her there.

In the days of King Arthur, a barge was summoned when it was time for someone to cross over the lake to the magical island of Avalon. This barge, which I imagine to be a roomy, flat-bottomed boat, was the vessel that transported the priestesses from the shores of Glastonbury through the mists to the island of the Goddess and back. This vessel of transition is also the means by which a menopausal woman finds herself journeying to her own inner world of Avalon. It is this same great, mystical barge, buoyed by a woman's willpower and inner strength, that returns her spirit to the place where it reigned before puberty and boys swept it away.

The appearance of this etheric, menopausal barge at the shoreline that separates the inner and outer world often comes as a surprise to many women, who may feel as though the vessel appeared out of nowhere to collect them. However, if you have read any stories about Avalon, you know that the magical vessel never arrives without being summoned. And so it is with a woman's body and menopause. Although the dispatching of the vessel may be carried out by her ovaries, it is the journeying woman's timekeeper who beckons it. And this timekeeper, this chronicle of her being, is a very precise instrument. Its ceremonious bidding to the menopausal barge is not a haphazard occurrence.

The arrival of the barge is a deliberate act gener-ated by the same life force that summoned her from the inner world when she journeyed through menarche-her first menstrual period.

Now scientists will claim that it is not as mystical as all that. They may say that menopause is a bodily function and nothing more. After all, the pause of menses is the direct result of ovaries and eggs dying off. It is the result of declining levels of estro-gen, progesterone, and androgens. Or else it is the result of surgery, or chemotherapy, or an autoim-mune disease or a bad environment, etc., etc., etc. But is it really? If we could keep the hormones flowing, could we keep the menopausal barge from coming? Could we keep the voyage to the wise-woman years at bay forever?

I don't think so. A woman's journey into menopause and the wise-woman years is not about atrophy at all. It's not about dying eggs or hormone levels, either. Although the decline of a woman's reproductive system is certainly a manifestation of menopause, the mid-life voyage itself is much more meaningful than that.

Menopause is really a journey of moving inward. It is about a woman turning her activity, her attentions, to the core of her very being. It's about seeking out that most sacred spot deep within the recesses of her heart, and rediscovering the divine nature of the Godlike, spiritual self that lives there.

The problem that most women have with making the menopausal journey inward is that by the time they reach their mid-thirties and early forties, they've forgotten that such a place exists. For the past quarter of a century they've practiced self-denial, self-control and self-discipline to the point of having very little self at all. They've lived for so long in the outward that their true nature has become little more than a faint memory.

And what is the outward? The outward is about children and husbands and careers and putting on with and putting up with. It is about being a social director, mother, and hostess for the world. It is about never, ever having time for oneself because laundry has to be done, and kids and husbands need attending, and there's a stack of papers from the office that need looking at. It's about all the things women think they have to do in order to be important.

A few years back I read that most first-born children believe that they have to be first at everything in order to be important. I thought that extremely odd. I immediately turned to my four-year-old, first-born and asked her, "Do you think you have to be first at everything to be important?" Without hesitating for a moment, she curtly replied, "Of course!" I was concerned about this and tried to explain to her that she was important, not because of her birth order, or how she placed in a contest, but because she was a child of God. And although I made a special note in my mind to keep reminding her of her innate value, I knew that the problem went much deeper than that. It was not an issue of being first-born, it was an issue of being woman-born. For even as I was resolving to denounce this fallacy, I was also diligently running myself into the ground trying to be first and best so that I, too, could be important.

It is this way for women of all ages. Somewhere along the way we learned that in order to be important we had to be first, or best or exceptional at everything. We've forgotten that we are daughters of God and that as such we have an intrinsic value no matter what we do. We pretend not to remember that we are the "beloved" and that in God's eyes we are always first and best. And so we insist on carrying double the load, just to have what we already own. We work outside the home as well as inside the home to show our mates and each other just how indispensable we are. We work nights and weekends and holidays. We work and we work and we work, just trying to be important.

I wanted to cry when I learned that, as a whole, females are much shallower breathers than males. It's as if we don't even feel entitled to take up air space on the planet. That's what the outward will do to a woman if she stays too long. Once she has given all that she has to give, the outward will convince her to give more, even if it means giving up breathing. That is why women break down around the time of menopause, not just physically, but emotionally and mentally. And when they sense the breakdown is near, the timekeeper of their soul summons the barge. It is time to go home.

But what about women who have had their ovaries and uterus removed? Does a surgically induced menopause mean that the barge has been summoned unwillingly? I don't believe so. For it is the soul's desire to go inward that brings about the disease of the reproductive organs in the first place.

The uterus, fallopian tubes and ovaries represent the ties that a woman has to the outer world. And a soul who intends to remain in the outward will immediately repair and heal any disease or infliction that is occurring in these organs. So, again, the summoning of the barge is most assuredly an act that is instigated by the woman's own desire to make the trip home.

I silently summoned the barge at age 35 after a dear cousin of mine died. My grief felt overwhelming at the time, and I began to lose weight quickly. At first I thought nothing of it, but I know now that the mechanism had been turned on. The vessel was definitely on its way. Within nine months an enormous ocean liner was at my doorstep.

Although often surprised by its appearance, most women welcome the sight of the barge and gladly step onto it once it arrives. For they instinctively know that in order to keep their spirit intact, they must remove themselves from the outward.

However, a few women are not quite as thrilled about making the journey inward. The menopausal boat pulls up and they scream "not yet," all the while scrambling for higher ground in the outward. Although their souls sent out the call that summoned the barge, they prolong stepping onto the vessel and going home because they see it as a death call. They are afraid to say good-bye to the outward for fear it won't exist without them, or out of fear it won't be there when they return.

One of the myths that keep a woman tied to the outward is that her children, her husband, and/or her career won't survive unless she is up to her neck in handling the endless, sticky details of their lives. But what women don't understand is that the detailed work of the outward is what will truly destroy them in the end. I have seen it in myself, and I have seen it in my friends. It is the seemingly small details that, like termites, gnaw away at our inner home until nothing is left but the kitchen sink.

In her book, *Women Who Run With The Wolves*, Clarrisa Pinkola Estes writes of a tale called "Sealskin, Soulskin," that is reminiscent of the menopausal journey home and what happens when women relinquish their souls to the outward. In the story, a sealwoman has her sealskin stolen by a lonely fisherman. The fisherman promises to give it back to her if she will live with him for seven years. The sealwoman agrees, and goes home with him. During the seven years, the woman and the man make a child, and the woman, though content enough with her life, becomes increasingly uncomfortable living in the outer world. Her skin becomes dry and parched, her eyelids start to peel, her hair starts to fall out (all signs of menopause). One night the child awakens to his parents arguing. It has been seven years and the sealwoman is demanding to have her sealskin back. "I want what I am made of returned to me," cries the sealwoman. The husband refuses to give his wife her sealskin back, for fear that she will leave him. The child goes back to sleep but awakens later in the night to the sound of the wind, and goes out into the dark. He comes upon his mother's sealskin and returns it to her. The sealwoman pulls on her sealskin, grabs her child and heads for the ocean. She breathes into the child's mouth three times and then dives deep into the waters. Together they swim until they are home with her family.

When I first read the segment where the seal-woman cries "I want what I am made of returned to me!", I felt a chill run through my soul. That is what the journey into menopause is about-having what we are made of returned to us. After years of living in the outward, which is a man's world, women finally want what they are made of returned to them. They want to be moist and tender, and still be of value. They want their skins and hearts back. They want to care for their children without being underpaid, underpriced, and underloved. Unfortunately for the sealwoman, and for us, we can't have it both ways. At least not yet. We still live in a world where testosterone driven people bring home the biggest steak.

What are women to do, then? What was the sealwoman to do? I can't help but think if the man had given his wife back her sealskin earlier, then she wouldn't have become so dried out and parched and utterly distraught in the first place. Maybe she could have taken small trips back into the ocean and still been able to live with her husband and child. Or maybe she should never have given up her sealskin to begin with. There are many solutions to this tale. But the point is that most menopausal women are past the point of hanging onto their sealskins, anyway. It is too late. They gave up their skins and their souls long ago. The best they can do is to retrieve them, and again, they can do that by going inward, by going home.

So what happens once the menopausal woman actually does get on the barge, which all women eventually do, whether they fight it off at first or welcome it with open arms? One of the first things a woman will notice, besides the barge itself, is the muscular little man who steers it. In Marion Zimmer Bradley's *The Mists of Avalon*, he is described by Morgaine as not one but as several little dark men, with hands "as hard as horn." In Jungian psychology, this man at the helm of the menopausal barge is referred to as the animus, a masculine figure that resides in every woman's psyche. The animus represents the hidden, masculine side of her nature. It is the aggression that rises up and rescues her from harm in the outer world. And during the menopausal journey, it is the dark, instinctual animus that will guide her barge safely home, if she lets it.

There is a certain type of surrender that happens when a woman lets the animus in her take control of her barge. It is not the same type of abandonment that occurs when she allows her husband or children or her career to take her sealskin away. This type of surrender is more of a relinquishment than a submission. The voyage across the lake to menopause can be extremely difficult-physically, emotionally, mentally, and spiritually-and a woman will need all the strength she can muster to make it to the other side. Seeking refuge in the power of her animus is a wise idea at this stage of her life. For once she has turned the controls over to her animus, she is able to focus more closely on the rituals themselves.

Another thing a woman notices once she settles in on the menopausal barge is that all types of ailments have begun to surface from the bottom of the lake. Thankfully, in the beginning, before full blown perimenopause (the most difficult stage of menopause) has arrived, these ailments are usually more bothersome than painful.

One of the most common complaints a woman may have at this time is that she is not sleeping well. She may not be a true insomniac, but she most assuredly knows that something is amiss in her cycle. Whether she finds herself waking up every morning at 4:00 A.M. or finds herself unable to drop off at all, the further a woman drifts away from the outer world, the harder it is to get eight straight hours of sleep.

I have read many books and talked with many physicians about this sleep issue. Some say it is a lack of estrogen, some say a lack of progesterone. Still others say it is the night sweats and daily stress that cause the interruption in sleep. But not everyone who has a hard time sleeping is experiencing night sweats, and since stress has been a part of most women's lives for many years, I find this explanation hard to swallow. Although the sleep changes may in part be caused by hormonal imbalances, I believe that the disturbance of a woman's circadian rhythms at this time is genuinely the result of something much deeper.

For it is at this time, when a woman is settling into the barge, that she starts to awaken to her inner surroundings. Just as her body is stirring at all hours, her soul is also beginning to stir. This sudden awareness feels odd to her at first, and is most unsettling. I can't help but picture Miss Clavel in the story of *Madeline*, robed in her full length white night gown sitting straight up in bed and proclaiming, "Something is not right!" But this is how it is for the menopausal woman. Her soul is proclaiming that something is not quite right with her life, and at the same time it is awakening her to the fact that she has started the journey inward to mend it.

Many physicians say that this lack of sleep is also the culprit behind a woman's fuzzy thinking during the early stages of menopause. Some women refer to this fuzzy thinking as a short-circuit type of clicking that goes off in their brains at odd times during the day or night. Other women complain of momentary memory lapses, or say they feel as though their minds have gone blank. But the clouded memory of a journeying woman is not a result of sleepless nights, for even women who are continuing to sleep well experience it. I believe that a menopausal woman's lack of mental clarity is a direct result of her desire to shut herself off from the outer world. It is simply another indication that she has taken off in the direction of home.

Another minor issue that may surface once a woman summons the barge, is the change in her weight. Many women find that the farther along they go on their journey, the harder it is to keep weight off. For other women, keeping weight *on* becomes a problem. These changes in weight are caused by fluctuating hormones and the body's need to either stockpile or pillage estrogen from fat cells.

Usually when a woman is gaining extra weight at menopause it is because her metabolism has slowed down in an effort to conserve every little bit of estrogen. And when a woman is losing weight rapidly, it is usually because she has an extremely high metabolism and her body is using every little bit of estrogen it can get a hold of, even if it means depleting what it can from fat cells.

Although I'm sure it is a heated topic in many circles, I believe it is better for a woman to put on a little extra padding as she makes the emotional journey inward than to be stuck in the middle of the menopausal lake without an ounce of estrogen to her name. And studies do show that women who are slightly overweight have fewer menopausal complaints than do women who are underweight.

In addition to weight loss and gain, there are some other physical symptoms that accompany this first sacred ritual of summoning and stepping onto the barge. Symptoms like menstrual irregularities, cramps, migraine headaches and dry skin. Thankfully, most of these ailments are brief and relatively minor, for once a woman has summoned the barge, she must then summon her strength in preparation for the following ritual-that of pulling down the mists.

THE SECOND RITE:

PULLING DOWN THE MISTS

EVEN IF A WOMAN IS somewhat indifferent to the ritual of the summoning of the barge, the commencement of the second rite, that of pulling down the mists, will most certainly get her attention. And rightfully so. This second ritual ushers in distinct physical changes in the female body that make a woman more mindful of her whereabouts in the grand scheme of things.

The mists themselves symbolize the veil between the inner and outer world of a woman's soul. They represent mystery and drama and a sort of nether-world drifting that clouds the view of both Avalon and the material world. The mists also represent a secret passageway to the Great Isle of her inner being, a place whose whereabouts only she knows. And the act of pulling down these mists represents a conscious effort on the woman's part to find that deeper, hidden meaning within her life.

One of the first and more obvious signs that a woman is in the process of pulling down the mists around her is that she, like the adolescent girl at the onset of puberty, begins to move through a lot of unpredictable behavior and emotions. Not so surprisingly, these mood swings mimic the same ones that she experienced at 12 when she was passing from the mists into the outer world. Only now she is expected to be more in control of the transitions, so much so that the very idea of bursting into tears or complaining about the physical ailments becomes shameful. This should not be so. And the pulling down of the mists is not a rite that a woman should do out of shame, nor one she should do out of a need to disappear from the outside world. It is a rite that she should perform out of her desire to direct her attentions to her inner world and concentrate more fully on what lies ahead.

This ritual can also be compared to the eight month of a woman's pregnancy when she is overwhelmed with a nesting instinct and feels as though she needs to rearrange the furniture. The journeying woman is restless and agitated at this point in the voyage, for she instinctively knows that there is little, if any, time left to make preparations for her trip inward. And so this act of pulling down the mists becomes the ritual that allows her to make these preparations efficiently and effectively.

The very idea of pulling down mists around oneself depicts seclusion and isolation, and in a nutshell, that is what this second ritual requires. With the exception of puberty, never will a woman feel more inclined to be alone than now. A friend was telling me that at the start of her menopausal journey she just wanted to find a cave to live in. We then speculated whether or not at some point in history women actually did hibernate during menopause. I haven't been able to find any data on it, but I can bet a number of women today would welcome the opportunity to do so.

In order for a woman to properly and securely pull down the mists around her, she must begin to make time for herself. And not just once or twice a week, but every day. Whether it's in the morning before her children rise, at lunch break, or in the evening after everyone else is asleep, a woman needs to have at least an hour or more to herself each and every day.

Finding time alone is not easy, though, especially when children and significant others are used to having a mother/wife at their beck and call. I have made a daily ritual of going into my office, which is located at the back of our house, every day from seven to eight o'clock in the evening to write. I feel that my seven and ten year old children and my forty year old husband should be able to entertain themselves for such a brief time. However, even as I write this paragraph, they are yelling questions to me through the locked door. My husband has even called me on the office line from the other end of the house to ask where the television remote is. I am considering getting an office away from the house with no phones. In the meantime, I must make do. For I know that any time away I can steal to be at peace with myself, which for me comes through writing, is time well invested.

Some other methods a woman may use to facilitate the ritual of pulling down the mists around her are reading, knitting, or taking a hot bubble bath. Prayer and meditation are also great for carrying out this sacrament of finding time alone.

One of my favorite rituals is writing in a journal. Keeping a diary came naturally to most of us during puberty, and many women still find pleasure in putting their feelings down on paper. There is a certain relief that comes in materializing the endless train of thoughts that tend to race through the mind during menopause. Expressing yourself in a journal is a way of validating and giving purpose to these thoughts. It also a way of spiraling inward, so that a woman can focus on herself, and redefine where she is on her voyage. The journal can then become a map of sorts to refer back to should she begin to feel lost in the mists of her menopausal symptoms.

An additional method that not only gives a woman time away from the outside world, but allows her to strengthen herself physically and emotionally as well, is exercise. There have been dozens of studies that prove that exercise reduces the symptoms of menopause. Certain exercises not only increase bone mass, but they improve memory, circulation, emotional well being, and they contribute to a better night's sleep. And one doesn't have to join an expensive health club to reap the rewards of a good workout either. Exercise tapes on everything from stair-stepping to yoga are available at the local video stores. If nothing else, one can always throw on a pair of tennis shoes and jog around the neighborhood.

How a woman chooses to pull down the mists is inconsequential, though, as long as it gets done. For it is extremely important that the pulling down of the mists should be executed while a woman is well enough to do it for herself, rather than having it done for her, and possibly to her, by outside forces. Often a woman heading into the menopausal years will run herself ragged and then, on a verge of a nervous breakdown, spend thousands of dollars and countless hours on a psychiatrist's couch trying to figure out what went wrong. If a woman elects to pull down the mists by her own hand, using her own willpower and energy, then she will feel much more in control of her journey.

One of my favorite passages about the mists that separate Avalon from the rest of the world is from *The Mists of Avalon.* In the book, the pulling down of the mists is performed by the priestess commanding the barge, and is executed shortly after the barge moves away from the shoreline. It is described in one scene as an act in which the Lady of the Lake must summon all her strength to perform:

> *"She stood still, rigid, locked into the tension of magic, then stretched out her arms, extending them full length, raising them high above her head, palms toward the sky. Then, with a swiftly exhaled breath, she brought them down-and with them fell the mists . . . ."*

This act of pulling down the mists, of shrouding oneself in darkness and seclusion, requires a great deal of faith from a perimenopausal woman. Faith that she will not get lost in the mists. Faith that she will eventually, at some point, reach the Great Isle on the other side of the lake. And most certainly, faith that she has the ability to transmute. Without faith, and a large dose of courage, this second ritual can quickly turn into a menopausal nightmare. It is very easy for a woman to let fear overwhelm her at this time, because as her hands go up to pull down the mists, the second thoughts about and remembrance of old lovers starts rushing in. The "Why haven't I's?" and the "Why didn't I's?" coupled with the increasingly difficult physical ailments are enough to freeze anyone in the moment. In fact, it is here that a lot of women (and men) get frozen or stuck in their lives. They refuse to make the transition through their mid-life crisis and end up wandering around aimlessly on the barge looking for the great isle of Avalon. But it is part of the mystery and magic of Avalon that one must ride through the mists in order to find it.

By their very nature, the mists that separate a woman's inner world from her outer world are dark, dense, and heavy, almost suffocating. This is a principal fear for a lot of women, and rightfully so. The sense of not knowing where one is headed, the loss of control, the feeling that some unseen monster or tragedy will jump out from around the bend can be terrifying. And these things I've described are actual menopausal feelings. I went around for months upon months waiting for something horrible to happen. I couldn't seem to get a handle on my anxiety, nor could I put it into words. And there are still times when I find myself lost in the mists of my inner and outer world and the fear seems overwhelming.

In the tales of Avalon, it is said that the mists were raised and lowered by a woman's magic. And in the outer world a woman's magic has always been equated with her beauty. I believe that much of the apprehension that menopausal women experience is a direct result of this. The anxiety of moving through the mists is really a fear of losing one's magic/beauty during the journey. Or, worse, fear that one never possessed the magic/beauty to begin with.

Therefore, as she pulls down the mists it is important that the menopausal woman keep reminding herself that her magic does not spring from her youth, it is her youth that springs from her magic. Youth is just a seasonal expression of a woman's true nature. It cannot and will not ever be able to define or encompass all that she is. Making that trip back to Avalon does not in any way diminish a woman's charm or magic or beauty. In fact, it is the trip itself that strengthens a woman's ability to captivate. And it is the journey inward that allows her to further hone the innate skill of attracting good into her life.

When I was in the early, fearful months of this ritual, and had not yet been officially diagnosed as being menopausal, I instinctively knew that I was going through some type of hormonal metamorphosis. I remember telling a family member that I felt as though I was a caterpillar, wrapping itself up in its chrysalis. It was a scary process. I knew that when all was said and done I would eventually come out a butterfly, but the very idea of wrapping myself up so tightly that I couldn't see or move or hear for months, or years, was terrifying.

But that is what a woman must do when she pulls down the mists around her. She must wrap herself up in her own skin to become the caterpillar in the cocoon. And this securing herself up in her own skin is what facilitates the menopausal process by temporarily closing the veil between her and the outer world.

For when the menopausal woman is snug in her cocoon, away from the sticky details of the outer world, she has only her own soul to listen to. She cannot hear the voices of the outer world, only of the inner world. And as she sails further into the mists, she sails closer and closer to the voice that was hers long ago. The one that demanded its fair share of the pie. The one that told the truth no matter how embarrassing it was to others. The one that was not afraid to sing out of tune in church or at birthday parties. The one that asked embarrassing questions because it needed to know. This is the voice she must now trust. That is the voice that looms in the darkness of the menopausal mists.

And this voice is how, when a menopausal woman is deep in the fog of her two worlds and too terrified to move, she will know that she is still headed safely for home. For when she is very still in the cocoon of her own moist skin, she can hear that voice calling to her from just beyond the shadows, reassuring her that she is almost there.

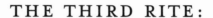

THE THIRD RITE:

THE GREAT INITIATION OF PERIMENOPAUSE

ONCE A WOMAN HAS securely pulled down the mists around her, she will often find that her uneasiness begins to worsen. The low level anxiety that was merely bothersome in the last ritual has quickly reached the point of outright panic, as hot flashes, night sweats, and depression start to set in. These symptoms, which are often referred to in the medical community as perimenopausal ailments, are what define the third ritual of the menopausal journey.

Up until the nineteenth century, when women were dying at the ripe old age of 50, these physical ailments were associated with a sort of old age dementia.

In the twentieth century, physicians discovered that these symptoms were actually a result of the deteriorating female reproduction system. Perimenopause ("peri" meaning perimeter) then became known as the time just before the pause of menses when the ovaries wind down and stop producing as much estrogen, progesterone, and androgens.

However, as we move into the twenty-first century, I believe that there will be a shift in the way women and their physicians view these perimenopausal complaints. Instead of being classified as ailments, I believe these symptoms will be known as the stimulus that transforms a woman from childbearer to bearer of wisdom. In the future, dry skin and sagging body parts will be seen as a sign that the great initiation of the wise-woman years has begun, and the pains that come in the form of night sweats, anxiety, and hot flashes will be known as the grand instigators of this initiation.

This expansive thinking will not, of course, lessen the discomfort of declining hormones or make the spiritual trip back to Avalon any easier, but it will bring about a greater understanding of this third rite and the significance of the symptoms that accompany it.

The onset of ailments that are attributed to the perimenopausal initiation usually start somewhere between a woman's 35th and 45th birthday. In general, most of the symptoms that reek havoc on a woman at this time are a result of the decrease in available eggs from her ovaries and the decline in circulating estrogen, progesterone, and androgens.

What often happens is that the lower levels of hormones will cause a domino-like effect that will permeate every part of a woman's system. For example, low estrogen levels often prompt a woman's adrenal glands to take over where the ovaries leave off by producing higher amounts of hormones. This increased response from the glands, along with spending too much time in the outer world, can send a woman spinning into adrenal exhaustion.

In addition to making a woman feel alternately tired and anxious, adrenal exhaustion can then produce problems with the entire endocrine system, including the hypothalamus, pituitary, thyroid, parathyroid, and pancreas. An imbalance in the hypothalamus often brings about night sweats, hot flashes, and insomnia, and an imbalance in the thyroid and parathyroid can lead to hyperthyroidism or hypothyroidism.

To further complicate things, low levels of estrogen aren't the only culprits behind the painful symptoms and illnesses of perimenopause. Actually, a change in any one of the hormones can throw the entire endocrine, and even the entire body out of sync. High levels of estrogen, commonly known as estrogen dominance, can cause menstrual flooding, cramps, and migraine headaches. Having too much or not enough testosterone can cause depression, loss of libido, irritability, and severe changes in the skin. Too little or too much progesterone often has the same affects.

Overall, perimenopause is a state of being unbalanced. And since the body is always seeking a state of balance, the overcorrection of putting out too much hormone versus not putting out enough, can leave a woman feeling as though she has been hit by a truck. Unfortunately, this phase of being in hormonal limbo can last a number of years.

Up until my own initiation into this stage, I believed menopause was a single event that happened to women in their early fifties and was over in a month's time. No one had ever told me, and I had never bothered to ask, about it being a process-one that can last up to ten years.

There has been much speculation about why the perimenopausal phase lasts this long. Why does it take a woman's body so much time to adjust? Why must the trip across the lake be such a slow one? One reason is that the ovaries don't just stop making hormones overnight. As noted before, the hormones, especially estrogen, go through periods where they surge, and the ovaries and adrenal glands put out twice as much as they usually do. Because the female body is estrogen dependent, the periods of surging hormones versus the periods of little to no estrogen at all tend to leave a woman feeling like a heroin addict needing a fix. And these shallow waters of the voyage versus the five feet tall waves brought on by the surges cause her body to constantly feel as though it is going somewhere, when in fact it is making very little progress across the lake.

Fortunately, this phase of feeling trapped and seasick in the middle of two worlds eventually builds up to a perimenopausal crisis and forces the barge in the direction of Avalon. This peri-menopausal turning point is the time when the water hits a boiling point, and the frustration that a woman has kept hidden over the last few decades spews out over the lake like Old Faithful.

As with all initiations, perimenopause then becomes a great instigator, a prompter of sorts. It becomes the fire under the feet, the needle in the side, the barking dog at a woman's heels that makes her get up and feverishly paddle for home. It becomes the giant tidal wave that eventually roars up and propels the barge toward Avalon. If it weren't for the crisis in this perimenopausal ritual, most women would be left floating in the dark mists forever and there would be no change.

My own initiation into perimenopause came one hot day in June when I found myself in the emergency room. I had been feeling tired and run down all week, but that Friday when I woke up I knew something was wrong. I couldn't breathe and thought I was having an asthma attack. A neighbor rushed me to the hospital where doctors ran two day's worth of tests and detected a floppy heart valve. I was given a beta blocker by my cardiologist and sent home to recover.

But recover I didn't. In fact, I got worse. I began to feel intermittently depressed and anxious. I was having memory lapses, and my periods were as erratic as my moods. It was at this time that I became certain that I was going crazy. After some prompting from my mother and with the recommendation from a close friend, I found a sympathetic endocrinologist who took blood samples and confirmed that my estrogen and progesterone levels were extremely low. He prescribed natural estrogen and progesterone made from soy by a compounding pharmacist, and within a month, I was feeling remarkably better, heart valve and all. I later read that fluctuating hormones can make the symptoms of my ailment—mitral valve prolapse—even more pronounced.

This is not to say that the initiation ritual of perimenopause can be skipped or lessened by starting on hormone replacement therapy. HRT was helpful in my case, but that isn't the way it is for every woman. I have talked with many women who say that HRT, even the natural forms, didn't help at all. Others say that they never felt like they were on the right dosage, and I have even found a few who said that hormones made them feel worse.

Choosing to use hormone therapy is not a decision that should be made lightly. It is a decision that should be made by a well-informed woman and a knowledgeable physician, and I stress the word "knowledgeable" here. Information that was doled out twenty, or even ten, years ago in medical school will not pass muster in the days of ever changing, ever evolving pharmaceutics.

There is a book by Gillian Ford titled *Listening To Your Hormones* which can be quite helpful to a women trying to make her way through the menopausal maze of HRT remedies. The book is full of information about hormone imbalances and lists most, if not all, of the options that are available to women who are having a hard time with perimenopause.

Again, however, it is important to remember that perimenopause is a ritual, a phase of a woman's life that must be walked through, not around. Even women who find complete relief from their symptoms through HRT or herbs must still pass through the initiation ritual.

On the other end of the spectrum from women who will try anything to get rid of the symptoms are the women who will try to deny the ritual all together. Like those who ran for higher ground when the barge arrived, a few negating souls still have a hard time believing that the menopausal voyage is under way. It's easy to do, especially when there are so many uninformed health care practitioners out there who are willing to play along with the phrase "oh no, you're much too young."

But the truth is that the menopausal voyage can begin at any age. If a woman is unsure, her first step would be to have her blood tested. But even then, the blood tests may state that she is not on the voyage when the wise-woman within her is screaming that not only has she started the journey, but she is halfway there. I firmly believe that any woman over 35 should have blood tests done periodically to determine her hormone levels. Although not inexpensive, the tests are painless, and there is simply no reason why a woman in her thirties or older should not have them done if she is experiencing perimenopausal-like symptoms. This means everything from backaches to insomnia should be investigated. And if a woman's regular physician won't do the tests, she needs to find one who will.

In addition to being the great instigator of change, the ritual of perimenopause lends a great deal to the evolution of a woman's soul and to her spiritual voyage back to Avalon. Like all great challenges, there are many lessons that come as a direct result of a woman's ability to actually complete this difficult ritual.

I believe that one of the most valuable disciplines a woman acquires during her passage through perimenopause is patience. Patience in moving through the pain, patience in not rushing the process, and patience in allowing herself the luxury of imperfection.

Someone once told me that patience is like a muscle. When you are stretching a muscle, it tears a tiny bit and then quickly repairs itself, and each time you stretch it, it tears a little less. Soon the muscle becomes very flexible and stretching farther distances becomes easier and easier. And so it is with patience. If a woman learns to stretch her patience during this initiation ritual, slowly pushing it beyond its boundaries, it will react like a muscle, coming back even stronger and more flexible the next time around.

Gratitude is another lesson that a woman acquires from perimenopause. Gratitude that the painful part of menopause is over may seem inconsequential at first. But there is a certain serenity and thankfulness that comes from being over any painful experience. This newfound gratitude after perimenopause allows a woman to appreciate all the things she had taken for granted in the outer world, and it allows her to sail more smoothly into the inner world. For in the inner world, nothing is taken for granted. This is why children always find such wonder in small, seemingly insignificant things. It is not just because they are seeing things for the first time, but because they instinctively know that there is joy in all things and all beings.

In addition to stretching her patience and reminding her of the importance of gratitude, perimenopause has a way of heightening a woman's senses in general. I have spoken with many women who felt an elated sense of awareness, that was, at first, extremely uncomfortable.

This odd sense of awareness began with "formi-cation"—a prickly feeling in the legs and arms that is quite common during perimenopause. It was this itchy-crawly feeling that seemed to stir their blood, and make them want to get up in the middle of the night and run around the block a couple of times. These same women said they later started noticing that the tingling feeling that accompanied their hot flashes also stirred their blood, giving them an almost quaking feeling. During this time they felt as if they were shedding their skins, or molting. Every nerve seemed to stand on its end, ready to burst through the outer layers of their being.

This pulsating of power that surges through the journeying woman at menopause reminds me of a sign that my endocrinologist has up in one of his rooms that reads "I'm not having a hot flash, I'm having a power surge!" And indeed that is what is happening.

Perimenopausal women are plugged into the universe, and the power switch has been flipped. Although uncomfortable, the initiating woman must continue to remind herself that her body will become accustomed to these unfamiliar feelings of power. And over time, she will learn to effectively harness the atomic energy that comes with being postmenopausal.

In the meantime, she must concentrate on moving through the painful ritual of perimenopause and on toward home.

THE FOURTH RITE:
THE QUEST FOR HOLINESS

THERE IS A NOTED PROVERB that states that success is a journey, not a destination. And so it is with menopause.

Although most every menopausal woman would rather move through the process as quickly as possible, it is important to remember that it is by the voyage, not the destination, that the fruits of the wise-woman years are harvested. Only by braving the rough waters of perimenopause can a woman truly know how strong her barge is. And only by experiencing the journey inward can she find the wholeness that she so desperately seeks. The fourth ritual symbolizes the gateway of a woman's journey inward to find that wholeness. It also marks the beginning of her attempts to reclaim that ever elusive soulskin.

Up until this time, the menopausal woman is sure that her incapacitating symptoms are the result of physical changes going on in her body, and she is confident that if she can just find the right dose of hormones, the rest of the voyage will be smooth sailing.

However, she soon finds that the relief that comes from quieting the physical symptoms of peri-menopause is only temporary. And the patches and pills that once seemed like a miraculous cure inevitably become the band-aid on the gaping wound of her soul as she pushes to find an even deeper meaning to her mid-life transformation. The journey inward then becomes more than just the quest to heal, it becomes the quest to make whole.

This quest to make whole, which is of course, also the quest to make holy, is further intensified as the woman peers into the reflection of her inner world. Although the waters have calmed a bit, they seem more muddled than ever. Have they always been this way she wonders, or is she genuinely noticing the murkiness for the first time? She closes her eyes and looks again. The lake becomes more obscure with every blink.

It is at this stage of the voyage, when women are still shrouded by the mists and contemplating their muddled, inner world reflection, that their outer worlds begin to unravel. It is often a time when children, and sometimes mates, are headed out the door for good while wives and mothers are left standing in the doorway holding the kitchen spatula.

Or this unraveling may appear when a woman's career and relationships are in a lull, and suddenly she finds that the glue of busy details that kept her outer world together for so long has mysteriously dissipated. Whatever the motive, the journeying woman finds that she has lots of time on her hands, and though somewhat unsettling, this lull allows her the time to further examine the view of her inner world.

Paradoxically, though, the harder she concentrates on her inner life, the worse things seem to get for her. The waters become stormy again, almost unmanageable. In addition to the physical and emotional symptoms, comes a profound spiritual uneasiness. The proverbial question of "Is this all there is?" hangs in her mind like a lighted billboard on an ever darkening horizon.

This spiritual uneasiness gives way to a feeling of panic rising in her soul, as she begins to feel even more anxious about her journey through the mists. She starts to second guess her internal exploration, all the while wondering if it might be better not to look so closely at her reflection. This is when every moment, every past experience of a woman's life, begins to be mentally and emotionally reproduced and scrutinized. Not so coincidentally, it also conveys a time when this examined inner life seems too painful to view.

I remember my mother telling me about a spiritual retreat she attended at a monastery. One of the processes involved the instructor walking down a line of visiting women and holding up a mirror for them to look into. Each woman was forced to stand in front of the group and look at her own reflection for five minutes. My mother related how uncomfortable it was to stare back at herself in the mirror for the allotted time while the others looked on, and she said that there were many women who turned their eyes away from their own reflection before their five minutes was up.

That is the way many women feel during this stage of menopause. It is too difficult for them to view their own inner reflection. It is too painful for them to see what they've become, and what they've disguised themselves as for so long. And it is even more painful to move through the viewing in front of witnesses.

It is at this crossroads that a woman must make a conscious commitment to look within, and to keep looking within, until the spiritual and emotional pain of the journey has healed. She must continue to see and to identify and to name what is at the bottom of her stormy menopausal lake. And most importantly she must continue to ride the barge out. For only by riding through the emotional storm can she restore the power that lies at the core of her soul, and only by restoring the power that lies at the core of her soul can she be made whole and holy.

However, the process of getting past the muddled, stormy menopausal waters and down into the core of her soul and bringing what she finds to light, is not an easy task for the apprentice.

First of all, there is an excess of emotional baggage threatening to sink her barge. And rather than toss it out, she mistakenly clings to it in hopes that it will save her should the barge sink. But that is a misconception. The baggage cannot save her. The baggage only represents her external connections to the outer world. And if the journeying woman is not careful, these external connections will become the anchors that ground her into the mists.

The mistake that women make of clinging to the bits and pieces of luggage is a common one. Like men, women tend to define themselves through external connections. These external connections, for men, often come in the guise of a career. For women, the connections, or pieces of baggage, are relationships. Ask a man who he is, and he will answer what he does—"doctor, lawyer, pilot." Ask a woman who she is, and she will answer who she is to other people—"mother, wife, sister." And even if it's the other way around, and a man answers "father" and a woman answers "politician," these are still not accurate portrayals of who they are.

These illusionary bits of emotional baggage that connect these women and men to the outer world are just reflections of where these men and women direct their energies. They are ties to what the subjects believe to be important, and of how they spend their days. They are not what connects them to God, and they do not represent what exists for them on a soul level.

So what does live in the deepest parts of the journeying woman's soul? What are the internal connections that define who she truly is? And how does she separate the external connections from the internal ones? The best way to proceed on this peeling back, this dumping of excess baggage and getting to the core to find out, is to thoroughly examine every part and parcel that is on the barge with her.

This means that the journeying woman must begin to focus in on, and consequently draw attention to, all areas of her life, from mothering to career, from past to present.

This is a very difficult process for the menopausal woman. For the more boxes and trunks she opens and examines, the more there is left to uncover and view. It will seem like a bad cosmic joke at first. Just when a woman thinks she's gotten to the core of her essence and examined all the bags, she finds that there is an entire mountain of suitcases that haven't even been touched.

Again, this is a painful procedure, for what a woman must disclose is often something that she has spent decades covering up. Hidden parcels filled with memories of sexual, physical, and emotional child abuse are discovered. Hat boxes stuffed with hurts and pains and grief of all forms suddenly become magnified in the light of the moon, and not only must be looked at, but must be sorted through and processed.

That is why, if one can possibly afford it, finding a good therapist who specializes in transitioning women is a must for completing this fourth ritual of the journey. If not, a good friend can be helpful. At the very least, one should keep a daily journal of dreams and thoughts. Dreams are the keys that open the doors of a woman's inner conscious, her Goddess-self. Dreams will also alert a woman to what areas of her life need to be examined first.

When I was feeling quite ill, a friend of mine sent the following piece to me from *The Mists of Avalon*:

> *"Hush, hush," he soothed. "You are weary and ill, you will feel better." He stroked her uncombed hair. "Sleep is the best medicine for your illness now, Igraine. And dreams are the true remedy for what ails you. I, who am master of dreams will send one to cure you." He stretched out his hand over her in a blessing and went away.*

How true to life this passage is. Dreams are not only the remedy for what ails us during this menopausal passage, but they are scripted directions on where we need to proceed in order to heal. They are truly the compass that points us in the direction of home.

A very wise female relative of mine was recanting her midlife passage and the vivid dreams she used to have at the time. One of the dreams involved her walking over to a casket and looking into it. Lying inside was a small girl dressed in a school uniform. The school girl in the casket opened her eyes and said "please don't let me die!" My relative took that dream to mean that she was to return to school and further her education. She did indeed go back and get her master's degree in social work, and was a wonderful therapist to me as I went through the most difficult part of my own transition.

One of the books that this same relative gave me during our talks included the tale of Psyche and her mother-in-law Aphrodite. In this tale, Psyche must complete several tasks for Aphrodite in order to win back her son, Eros. One of these tasks involves the sorting of millions of seeds. The job of sorting the seeds overwhelms Psyche and she immediately wants to give up and drown herself in a nearby river. Instead, she falls asleep and a colony of ants arrive to help her sort the seeds. By the time that she awakens, the task is complete.

The seeds in this story of Psyche remind me of the endless number of decisions and choices that a woman must make on a daily basis. Although decision-making has always been a part of her life, there is something about the time of menopause that makes even the most minor decisions seem overwhelming. Maybe it is being on the barge in between two worlds, or maybe it is the obscurity of the mists that clouds her judgment. But for whatever reason, the sorting of the endless choices and dilemmas becomes an almost insurmountable task.

Like Psyche, many women would rather escape into a river of alcohol and drugs than deal with the endless decisions and quandaries that plague them during menopause. In this case, it is again best to do what Psyche eventually does and wait them out. This doesn't necessarily mean that a woman needs to stick her head in the sand or ignore the problems, which is truly what she does when she turns to drugs and alcohol. But the old cliché of "sleeping on it" certainly goes a long way when a woman is faced with an onslaught of life-changing decisions.

This philosophy of sleeping on it, or waiting it out, goes against the grain of many women who have an innate desire to make a snap decision about anything and everything that comes along. Which is why they often feel so overwhelmed at the time of menopause. But the truth is that most decisions need not be made in a split second. And waiting until help arrives is often the simplest and wisest choice of all. Keep in mind, too, that help doesn't have to come from an outside source. In fact, it often comes from the tiny bits of intuition that spring up from a woman's soul only after she's given her intellect a chance to rest.

In the story of Psyche, the tiny bits of intuition come in the form of ants. When I first read how the ants came and assisted her in sorting the seeds, I thought it was odd. Then I realized how unique these tiny creatures are. Ants are the smallest of workers, but they are also quite strong. An ant can carry more than one hundred times its size and weight. It is also diligent and persistent in accomplishing its goal, and that part of the woman's intuition is what is needed for her to make her choices wisely and proficiently.

Another process that a woman can enact to help her in the sorting of seeds and choices, and more importantly, to help her decide what emotional baggage needs to be tossed overboard, is to break her life down into cycles, or phases, and inspect them one by one. She can easily accomplish this by making a list of all of her outstanding memories from childhood to recent years. Once she has made the list, she should then assign an emotion such as fear, love, hate, jealousy, etc., to each one. This means of identifying and naming each memory will enable her to define a pattern of emotions in her life.

Putting a name to the repetitive patterns of dramas and emotions is a necessary process. For when a woman names something, she gives voice and validity to the power it had over her. This acknowledgment also allows her to take responsibility for the excess baggage she has accumulated over the years. For only after she has conceded to her role in creating and carrying the baggage, can it be thrown overboard.

In naming these patterns, the menopausal woman will also find herself amazed at how circular her life has been. That is how it is for all of us. We perceive that our lives are linear, but in viewing the situations from a perspective, we see that the emotional dramas in our lives are like boomerangs that keep coming back. Like a coil curling around and around, we tend to make circles around the same old situations and circumstances. The plights and scenery of our lives may change as we age in years, but the underlining core of our lessons remains the same.

An additional tool a woman can use in getting to the core of her soul and ridding herself of excess baggage is forgiveness. Forgiveness for oneself as well as for others. When done with sincerity, forgiveness becomes the Excalibur of the inner world. It will cut through layers of pain and hopelessness faster than any other weapon a woman will carry. And although one doesn't have to forgive in order to let go, it certainly speeds up the healing process.

A good example of this might be a woman who has been violated at some point in her life and continues to embrace this violation and the idea of herself as victim. Once she allows herself to forgive the trespasser, she immediately releases the baggage connected with being a victim.

Unfortunately, forgiveness is not always that easy, especially if a woman has spent decades defining herself as a victim. Using forgiveness to crack the mold of eternal prey requires a woman to allow herself a certain amount of vulnerability. Again, she must have faith that the releasing of excess baggage will not leave her open to additional pain. She must trust the voyage and she must be willing to call on the inner wise-woman to protect her on her quest.

Judith Viorst wrote a book called *Necessary Losses: The Loves, Illusions, Dependencies and Impossible Expectations that all of Us Have to Give Up in Order to Grow,* that sums up the quest for holiness in its title. For in order to be made both whole and holy, a menopausal woman must stand erect at the edge of her barge and throw overboard all the illusions, dependencies, and impossible expectations of herself as well as those of others. She must rid herself and her barge of all that she is not in order to find her way home.

In essence, I believe that this fourth ritual is truly a ritual of remembrance. Remembrance of the ageless wisdom that lies buried at the core of every woman's soul, and remembrance of a woman's divine place in the universe. If only a woman can call up this remembrance and look to the Goddess within, she will find that, like Dorothy in the *Wizard of Oz,* she was both holy and home all along.

THE FIFTH RITE:

BATHING IN THE HEALING WATERS

THE LIBERATION FROM emotional baggage drastically changes how a woman views the remainder of her journey. Although she may still not feel completely whole, the sorting of seeds and ousting of skeletons has calmed the menopausal storms, and the barrage of ailments have, for the most part, lost their punch. The fear of being out of control has also eased its grip on the menopausal woman, and at last she is able to look into the water and see a clear picture of who she is.

The surrounding water reflects back a truer, sharper picture of a woman's feminine wisdom and spirit. Unlike the murky seas that raged around her during the Initiation ritual, this water reflects a purifying, cleansing image of the menopausal woman. As she ponders this new image, she sinks even deeper into her subconscious, inner world in an effort to further soothe and heal her psyche. She is now ready to perform the ritual of bathing in the healing waters.

Carl Jung wrote often of the symbolic ties that water has to the psyche and the subconscious. In fact, the symbolism of water as a healing and purifying agent both physically and spiritually, goes back as far as history is recorded. There are many verses in the Bible that refer to water, the most significant being John the Baptist's use of water to immerse and spiritually initiate his followers. Jesus was reported to have walked on water, a symbol of his ability to conquer the psyche. Seasonally, water encourages growth and rebirth among the plant kingdom; the spring rains stimulate the flowers, and grass and trees begin anew.

So it is with the menopausal journey, when a woman finds herself immersed in the clear, calm, healing waters of her inner world. She discovers a certain newness, a spiritual, physical and mental rebirth of sorts. The water itself may come in the form of her own tears, as she realizes that she is still subjected to fluctuating hormones. But the tears that flow now are of a cleansing nature, unlike the disparaging ones that plagued her during the early perimenopausal phase.

If a woman steadies herself against her barge and looks even farther ahead, beyond the healing waters, she will see the green land of Avalon. The Great Island becomes the closure of the seemingly endless journey, a finish line to mark the completion of the universal circle of life. It is this completion that will renew and further heal the menopausal woman after her long journey across the seas. Like a mandala, a circular figure that symbolizes healing and universal totality, the endless circle of land returns her to her beginnings, fulfilling her hunger for wholeness and completion.

During one of the most difficult times of my perimenopausal phase, my six year old son brought home a mandala he had made at school. The bottom of the picture read:

"The Mystic circle, simultaneously representative of sound, light, color, form, rhythm and harmony. Why create a Mandala? Because it has a calming and relaxing effect on the mind and body, thus focusing and strengthening the will to heal."

Years later, the drawing still hangs on my refrigerator door as a symbol of menopausal wholeness.

And so the journeying woman, now in the early stages of healing, is prepared to move into acceptance. This ritual of acceptance brings about a reconciliation with the self. This reconciliation, or joining of the inner and outer worlds, consequently ushers in a new level of spiritual awakening for most women. As the waters around the barge become smoother and clearer, so does the divine mind. And in place of the excess baggage, the rejuvenated spirit bubbles forth. Being inspirit, the journeying woman truly becomes an inspiration to herself and to others. Her creative energies are readying themselves for the crone years, when she will sprinkle them over the planet in a burst of postmenopausal zest. But for now, they will continue to quicken in the core of her soul.

This ritual of healing is a time of revelation in which a woman discovers her spiritual powers, and though still somewhat of an apprentice, begins to experiment with them. She may challenge her previous religious beliefs, vigorously questioning the doctrine she so faithfully followed before her transition (doing so, not out of a sense of irreverence, but out of the desire to uncover all that is not sacred in her life). Or it may be just the opposite. A woman who had tossed her spiritual beliefs overboard during the traumatic perimenopausal transition, fishes them out of the clear water and re-embraces them. However she decides to perform this ritual, the menopausal woman is sure to be regrouping and arranging her new found creed in ways she never thought possible.

This regrouping and rearranging gives a woman a revitalized sense of purpose and self-confidence as she once again learns to accept and see herself, her body, with the same relentless joy she did in her adolescent years. Like the sacred Grail, her round, robust hips and stomach suddenly become a chalice filled with great divinity. Her plump, fleshy thighs become inexplicably sexy and feminine. Her thick forearms turn into pillars of great strength. The menopausal woman transforms into the picture that is so often depicted in the paintings of rich woman in the middle ages— rotund, buxom, hearty, unabashed. She is now ready to wear the menopausal badge with pride.

This new stage of self-acceptance is not only healthy for a woman, but it is mandatory if she is going to make it the last leg of the voyage. For if she arrives at this stage still unready to accept the true and whole picture of who she is, than she will inevitably fall back into the dark mists, never to make it to Avalon.

This ritual is also the time when a woman finds *unacceptance* in the way she was formally treated by the outer world. She is no longer willing to put up with the dirty dishes and clothes on the floor. She is no longer willing to accept being told what to do by her subordinates, nor is she willing to let others take the credit for what she has accomplished. It's as if the moment the mists cleared, she is suddenly seeing the world for the first time. And perhaps she is. Her world has been clouded for many years now, veiled with too many responsibilities and too little appreciation. So she may, for now, continue to hold back her gifts and her time from the world until she has regained her balance again. Although no longer clouded in the mists, she may also continue to isolate herself from the outside world, and for a short period of time she may neglect her relationships.

Sadly enough, few women or men recognize this part of the ritual, of withholding one's gifts, as being temporary. Women who haven't completed the journey and don't yet bear the wisdom of the crone (who knows how to share her gifts appropriately) may feel guilty in their desire to withhold their energy and contributions. And mates and friends may feel as though the woman has deserted them all together. Fortunately, this ritual, like all the other rituals, will pass, and with the crowning of the crone the woman will once again share herself with the outer world.

In addition to revealing new insights into her worth, the cleansing ritual has brought about a new sense of integrity for the voyaging woman. Integrity in that the woman now has a clearer picture of the rights and wrongs of the world. Although not quite ready to speak the truth as it needs to be spoken, she most assuredly has a more vivid picture of it than she did during her childbearing years. Truth becomes very important to a woman at this phase. For once the vapors of the mists have departed, and the freshness of the healing waters have revealed the truth, the lies that have impaled themselves in the journeying woman's life are exposed in the brilliance of the healing sun.

This stark unveiling of the truth and lies of her outer world is a direct result of the sense of completeness that she is experiencing as she nears the end of her voyage. The circle, the mandala, the vision of The Great Isle just ahead of her, has brought her back to wholeness. And in this wholeness she finds honor and reverence where there once was shame and disrespect. The sight of her perfect and completed reflection in the water, coupled with the knowledge that she is about to step onto the sacred ground of her own inner-being, instills a tremendous sense of self-confidence in the journeying woman. She is aware of her wholeness and no longer needs companionship to feel completed. Therefore, she is quite selective about who she allows to accompany her the rest of the voyage. Anyone who threatens to compromise this newfound wholeness quickly finds themselves following the fate of excess baggage.

Clarity also becomes very important to a woman at this phase. Now immersed in this new sense of integrity, the menopausal woman discovers a sort of mental and spiritual clarity that she never knew she had. The clouded memory and forgetfulness of perimenopause, having been washed away with the storms, is immediately replaced in the journeying woman's intellect by an even greater source of wisdom. This new element of wisdom filters out any leftover feelings of confusion and further clears her vision of Avalon and her inner world. During the later stages of this ritual, many women start to feel as if they have developed an almost telepathic awareness, and indeed they have. For a woman's intuition, with the exception of the short period after she gives birth, will never be as strong as it is now.

Several theories abound as to the origin of the sudden influx of intuition that a woman acquires as her menstruation cycle winds down. One conjecture is that certain hormones (specifically the follicle stimulating hormone, FSH, and the luteinizing hormone, LH) which are extremely high during the menopausal years, do a sort of rewiring of the brain, heightening its awareness.

Another speculation is that the brain is exercising and flexing sections that had been dormant before menopause. So, in lieu of relying mainly on the left, or logical hemisphere of the brain to make decisions, the woman also begins using the right, or intuitive hemisphere.

An additional philosophy, (one that will be further discussed in the following ritual of Holding the Blood Within) is a belief that has been held in mystic circles for centuries. Its analysis is that a woman grows wiser in her menopausal years because she is no longer menstruating and is now holding the wise, life-giving blood within.

Whatever the science, or speculation, behind these lines of thought, a woman does indeed become more enlightened and opened to new ways of thinking during these later stages of her menopausal voyage.

And so the journeying woman, growing wiser by the years, sails on toward Avalon. Having summoned her barge, wrapped herself in mists and isolation, suffered the pains of initiation, made the quest for holiness, and experienced the healing waters of the great lake, she has completed the first five rituals of menopause, each of them just as difficult as the one before. At this point, she finds herself within inches of being one with her inner world. She can see, smell, taste, and touch the core of her soul. She is almost home.

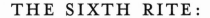

THE SIXTH RITE:

HOLDING THE BLOOD WITHIN

DURING THE SIXTH RITUAL, the journeying woman's barge arrives at its destination—the Great Isle of Avalon. And so she steps out onto the land, the mandala of her wise-woman years, and the circle closes for good. The accumulation of all that she has experienced over the last decade has come to a climax. She is now at the inlet of the next major phase of her life and will spend her last few days as childbearer preparing for her years as crone.

She finds this new land steady and solid beneath her feet, and the air fresh and liberating. She is completely absorbed with her newfound inner wisdom. Her spirit sores as she revels in the new sights and feelings that pulse through her heart and mind, for at last she has made it to the core of her soul to refresh and replenish all that the outer world has taken away. She is now free to dance among her people, to speak her own tongue, to be soft and tender and strong.

In the present day world, Avalon, which was actually named Annywfen by the Celtics, is not an island or even an exact destination. However, relics from the tales of the mystical land, along with the ruins of the Glastonbury Abbey, can still be found in Sommerset, England. The small town of Glastonbury, which is where one would have gone to summon the barge, surrounds the relics. Just on the outskirts of this small town on a large hill stands a 500 foot tower, or Tor. It is said that this sacred tower was where the priestesses of Avalon celebrated their holy days. And it is here, to the internal tower of her soul, that the menopausal woman also goes to celebrate her last menstrual cycles.

Like the women of old, she will celebrate her holy/wholly days in the interior chambers of the Tor, the tower of her own inner being. She will stay in the tower and on Avalon until she is ready to be crowned crone, or has been without a menstrual period for a year. It is here that she will be reunited with the wise-woman and the wise-child of her essence. It is here that she will have her soulskin returned to her and become moist again. And it is here that she will nourish herself, and learn to nourish others appropriately. She may still experience an occasional hot flash or other menopausal symptom, but for the most part, the journeying woman is feeling strong and rejuvenated.

From this point forward, the woman's menstrual blood/spirit, which has been cyclically given to the world for the past thirty some odd years, will be held within. This does not mean that she will not share her spirit with the outer world anymore. In fact, it is just the opposite. For once a woman masters the ritual of holding the blood within, she intuitively knows when to release her spirit and gifts to the world and when not to. She learns this from the wise-woman who she is now one with. And the wise-child, who she discarded long ago, is also, once again, by her side.

Much has been written about the wise-woman who resides within the feminine spirit, but little has been said about the wise-child who is her companion. The wise-child, as mentioned in the introduction, is that demanding, somewhat self-centered, and very self-empowered preadolescent girl that used to rule a woman's heart. She was left behind years ago when the woman grew up and married the world and all of its busy details. The wise-child/wild-child has a very strong presence in the postmenopausal woman's life. She is the one who demands that the sealskins be returned this very minute, and she is the one who says "NO!" and means it when things become too hectic in the outer world. She is the Pippi Longstocking of a woman's inner world. Like the animus, the male guide that accompanied the woman through perimenopause, this wise-child is the muscle behind a crone's power. If it weren't for the wise-woman's gentle nature and wisdom to balance her, the wise-child might, perhaps, make life unbearable for all those around the postmenopausal woman with her constant demands. But again, the postmenopausal woman has the wise-woman to balance the demands and harness the energy of the wise-child.

Although the cessation of her menses is a very liberating time for a woman, it can also be a time for grieving as the woman waves farewell to her childbearing years forever. This can be especially traumatic for a woman who yearned to bear a child and didn't. And even if she didn't want children, or had the amount that she wanted, hidden away in the tower of her inner being, a woman may begin to have second doubts. She finds her maternal instincts suddenly, and many times unexpectedly, beginning to rally as she finishes out her last menstrual periods. The biological clock has more than just ticked away, it has exploded in her heart like a time bomb. But like all of the losses we must endure, not only as women, but as human beings; this is a necessary loss that must be grieved. And it is the wise-woman within who comforts the journeying woman and allows her to grieve for the children that will come through her no more. It is also the wise-woman who will point out to her that although she will no longer be creating children, there are many other life-giving gifts she has left to bestow on the world. Gifts that she will learn to cultivate and harvest during the following ritual.

And so the woman's last menstrual cycle comes and goes on the isle of Avalon. Two, three, maybe even six months pass, and suddenly the woman realizes she has had her last period. As the year passes and she continues to hold the blood within, she becomes electrically charged with power. She finds that she is sharper mentally, physically, and spiritually than ever before. New ideas, new projects are popping into her head left and right. The depression lifts, the anxiety passes, and for the most part, all is well with her world.

Although there is no set amount of time that a woman is destined to stay on Avalon, most women start to remember and long for the outer world somewhere in the first year after their period stops. It's as if they suddenly wake up and remember that they left something simmering on the back burner. This is when the menopausal moth emerges from the chrysalis as a butterfly. The woman steps out of her tower and looks toward the lake. It is beautiful and safe there, in her inner world, yet she knows that she must return to the outer. She feels strong, having been marinating in her own juices and power for quite some time now, and is confident in her ability to live in the outer world, again.

The woman has learned many lessons and developed many talents while on the Island of Avalon, one of the most prominent being the ability to speak the truth. During the healing ritual, the journeying woman saw and knew the truth, but it is during this ritual of holding the blood and the power within, that she learns to speak it like it has never been spoken before. For there is no truth like the truth that spouts from a postmenopausal woman's mouth. I am reminded of my grandmother, who at the age of 82, will stand up and tell it like it is until it hurts. My mother, who is 62, and has been soft-spoken most of her life, is quickly becoming the same way.

It's shameful how we, as childbearing women, shy away from the truth. We first learned to do it when we entered puberty, as if power and sexuality were something to be embarrassed about. We conveniently left important topics like our menstrual blood and budding breasts out of conversations. Then we pretended not to notice that we were smarter, taller, and faster than all the boys on the block. By our early twenties, we knew better than to outdo our dates/mates. In our thirties and forties, we were so busy wildly spinning our energy in an effort to prove our worth that we couldn't recognize the truth if it smacked us in the face. So by the time we are entering menopause, we have ridden in the back seat of life so long that we have forgotten the truth all together. It is only after we have travelled to the land of Avalon and retrieved our amulet of power that we remember. And then we have the wise-child, back with a vengeance, who not only demands that we remember the truth about ourselves, but demands that we speak it loud and clear.

This voice empowerment that women develop as they cease their menses comes as a surprise to the outer world, and is often considered to be a result of being old, crotchety, senile and "out of sorts." While mature men, who have held the power of voice for most of their lives, continue to be referred to as commanding, assertive, and confident. It's a double standard for sure, one I hope will change as we become a more Goddess-friendly planet.

Another weapon a woman arms herself with in an effort to remain strong in the outer world, is an intolerance for injustice. As a maiden or childbearer, a woman may have remained silent about the injustices placed on her and those around her, but once she enters the wise-woman years, she develops a tenacious intolerance for injustices or bias of any kind. No longer will she stand by and idly watch as children are abused or friends disrespected. In fact, she has an innate ability to cut through and disclose everything from simple rudeness to out and out treachery. This ability and the desire to follow through with it comes as a direct result of her remembrance of the truth. For not only does she recognize the truth in herself, she recognizes the truth and power in others. This truth extends from her fellow human beings down into the plant and animal kingdom and back to Mother Earth herself. This is why women in their crone years are so abundantly giving of their time and energy; they are able to recognize the divinity in every living thing.

One of the last and most important weapons a woman takes back into the outer world is her ability to say "no" and mean it. It is while on the Isle of Avalon that she learns to tout the phrase, "What part of 'no' don't you understand?" This task of speaking the word "no" is something that women have been struggling with since the time they first tried talking back to Daddy. What female wasn't taught that polite girls never argue, or that nice girls did as they were told? It's no wonder that men are confused about whether women really mean "no" or not. Of course they mean "no." It's just that society has made it incredibly difficult for them to speak it.

Although my own parents encouraged me to speak my mind and tell the truth as I saw it, I still have a hard time telling people "no." For years I volunteered at more organizations than I could count on both hands. It's as though I had the letters "y-e-s" written across my forehead. In fact, it wasn't until I hit perimenopause and spiritually and physically crashed that I realized that when you say "yes" to others and don't mean it, you say "no" to yourself. And I might still be saying "yes," if it weren't for the wise-child in me screaming out whenever I am asked to do something that isn't in my best interest. It is the wise-woman who also steps in at this time and decides whether the tasks we are being asked to do are appropriate for us. She knows, even more so than the wise-child, when we are being pushed way beyond our limits, and she knows, too, when we should give in and agree to the task that is being asked of us.

And so the journeying woman, having empowered herself with the strengths of Avalon, is ready to step back onto the barge and return to the outer world. She embodies the wise-woman and wise-child within her, and she is absolutely crackling with energy and power.

Yet, there is one last sacred ritual that a menopausal woman must partake in, and that is "The Crowning of the Crone."

THE SEVENTH RITE:

THE CROWNING OF THE CRONE

THE TERM "CRONE" HAS received a great deal of unfavorable notoriety over the years. For centuries, the expression was used to describe a woman's appearance rather than her ability to think and act on her feet. Characterize a woman as a crone, and people would conjure up a picture of an old, decrepit, prune-like grandmother with a sour look on her face. Or they would assume you were referring to a witch, a term which has also received its share of negative publicity.

This fallacy of a crone being associated with old age originated in centuries past, when women who had achieved the status of crone did so without the help of modern medicine and proper nutrition.

Before the 1900s, women didn't live many more years past the age of menopause. And if they did, they tended to look much older than they actually were. One might also think that this is how the term "crone" became associated with death. But in fact, the ties between death and the crone originated from the followers of the Great Mother Goddess who believed that the crone had the ability to both restore and take away life.

Thankfully, times are changing, and for the most part, the word "crone" is now accurately being used as a synonym for a woman who not only embodies postmenopausal wisdom, but shares it with the world. It is the time when the wisdom and healing of a woman's menopausal journey quickens in her heart, and her desire to share all that she has learned drives her back to the outer world. And so, just as the maiden years symbolized the time when a woman gave birth to herself, and the childbearing years the time when she gave birth to others, the crone years symbolize the time when a woman gives birth to the planet by sharing all that she has learned.

This seventh, and last, ritual of the voyage, begins when the postmenopausal woman steps off of the island of her inner world and back onto the barge. Again, the menopausal barge represents the strength of a woman's psyche and her ability to ride across the waters of emotion without sinking. The barge is much stronger now, having made two trips across the lake (one during menarche when she first journeyed to the outer world, and of course the most recent one, when she journeyed from the outer world back to Avalon). Fortunately, this third trip is quite different than either of the other two. Unlike the first two trips, when the waters of the lake were murky and rough, the trip back to the outer world is soothing to the woman's soul. The postmenopausal woman is more confident and self-assured; she knows these waters and she knows her barge. The journey then becomes an expedient one, and she arrives back on the shores of her outer world almost immediately.

A woman is officially crowned a crone the moment she proactively reenters the outer world, and begins sharing her ageless wisdom and healing powers with the planet. The ceremonious crowning of a crone usually goes unnoticed by those in the outer world, but back on the island of Avalon the wise-woman and wise-child are both celebrating this joyous event. For this crowning symbolizes a blending of two worlds. At last the inner world of the woman's soul is spread freely out onto the planet in the form of spiritual gift-giving, and the journeying woman earns the title of Goddess and Crone.

It is important to remember that one doesn't have to have lived to be 50 to be considered a crone, though. Crones come in all ages and sizes. I've known women who have embodied the postmenopausal wisdom of the crone by the time they were 30, and I've known women who were 70 and still hadn't achieved it.

Just because a woman has journeyed to the inner world of Avalon and had her last period, doesn't mean she has reached the status of crone, either. Being officially, or unofficially, crowned a crone means being ready to return and serve the outer world as Mother Goddess. It signifies that a woman is willing and able to share her wisdom, not only with the other women of her tribe, but with the men as well. And it is with the authority of the crone that the woman returns to the outer world to reseed the planet and spread what she has learned with all living creatures.

Mother Teresa was probably the best known crone. Her name and memory is synonymous with the word service. She personified the Mother Goddess in a way that few women have. She started out by comforting one man on the streets of Calcutta, and ended up comforting a planet of men, women, and children. What made her a such a wonderful example of crone wisdom? I believe it was her willingness to serve. Not her ability or how many she actually did comfort and serve, but her willingness to attempt the task. She wasn't afraid to reach out to the dying and she wasn't afraid to reach out to the living. It was second nature to her. But we don't all have to be Mother Teresas in order to embody the Goddess. We only have to be willing to serve our tribes.

Another, perhaps lesser known but nonetheless genuine crone, was my great-grandmother. When I was a young girl, I loved to watch this woman, who we called "Fat Mamma," feed the chickens on her farm. She was a short, stout woman with thick fore-arms and strong, muscular legs. Her apron would be filled with seeds, and every few steps she took, she would reach into her apron and grab a fistful of feed and throw it haphazardly out to the chicks. Fat Mamma embodied the crone, and she not only nourished the chickens but she nourished the minds of her family as well. This is what being a crone is all about; it means reseeding the planet and feeding the younger "chicks." It means bring-ing back what you learned on your journey and tossing it all over the planet.

Actually, this willingness to serve is second nature to most women. In fact, the majority of volunteers at any given organization are women. What stops some women from achieving the status of crone in their latter years, though, is their inability to differentiate between being of service, which means to contribute to the welfare of others, and being subservient, which means to be useful in an inferior capacity. What often happens is that a woman is so burned out from being *used* in an inferior manner, that she rebels against being *of use* to others in any capacity. This type of thinking is a major factor (along with decreasing hormone levels) in a woman's midlife depression and anxiety.

An additional element comes in to play for women who have not been employed outside of the home. There is often a let down period that dominates a woman's moods when the children leave home. On one hand, the postmenopausal woman is ecstatic to see her offspring fly, and on the other she finds it lonely sitting on an empty, eggless nest. She is glad to be rid of the busyness that comes with raising children, but at the same time she feels as though a hole has been left in her heart. And indeed it has been. However, this is the time when being of service to the community can not only permanently fill that hole, but can expand her heart as well. At this time, a woman who has achieved the wisdom of the crone hears the calling of her tribes, her community, and steps up to the challenge. She either obtains a paid, creative position, or she volunteers her time to the many agencies who would love to benefit from a wise-woman's ways.

As crones, women become the butterflies who have not only emerged from their chrysalis, but have taken flight and are soaring across God's garden. They are the magnificent creatures with strong, colorful wings that pollinate the land. Their long, thin, mystical antennas alert and navigate them to where they need to volunteer and whom they need to serve. This is the time for women to hone their skills and seek out new ones. Their wisdom is at its peak now, and they need to share it with whoever is willing and intelligent enough to listen. Unfortunately, our culture is not as aware of the wisdom of the crone as it should be. There is still a stigma against the aged, especially women.

But the time has come for America, and cultures like her, to finally acknowledge the wisdom of its aging population. As we pass into the next century, the majority of the population will be over the age of 55. In fact, there will be 50 million postmenopausal women living and breathing on this great planet by the year 2005. Never has the planet been so ripe to absorb the knowledge from those who will be holding the blood in the twenty-first century. And we, as crones, must not let Mother Earth down. We must not let each other down.

The crones of our land must not back down off their thrones of wisdom. They must exchange their rocking chairs for pedestals, and their knitting needles for scepters. It is time to acknowledge the wisdom of the crone years and be proud to wear the title. It is also time that postmenopausal women not only envision and speak the truth, but that they actively seek out the truth in everything they do.

Most importantly, the crones of our land must take up storytelling. For true wisdom can never be harnessed and experienced until it is shared. We must bear witness to each other's journeys, and we must tell what we know to all who will listen. Young maidens need to know what to expect of their own menopausal journey to the inner world, and they need to be warned of what happens once they give their sealskins away. Young boys, too, need to be taught the power and wisdom of the Goddess and crone. They need to be shown how to respect and appreciate a woman's intuitive nature. And these things can only be rightfully shared by a woman who has completed the seven sacred rites of the menopausal voyage.

I believe that to perform this sacrament of storytelling is to truly experience the most sacred and holy of all seven rites. For when a crone tells what she knows, truthfully and with an open heart, she becomes the mandala, the healing, completed circle for her sisters. She becomes not only a storyteller, and bearer of wisdom, but she becomes the story itself.

And so now our journeying woman is at the end of her voyage. She has completed the seven sacred rites. She has embraced the internal world within and returned to the shores of the outer world, not as childbearer, but with the authority and power of the crone. She has forever become the storyteller and the story. She is, truly, whole and holy. She is feminine wisdom at its peak. She is the culmination of Eve, and Mary, and the Great Goddess within. She is, truly, all that The Great Divine created her to be.

POSTSCRIPT:

CELEBRATING THE CROWNING OF THE CRONE

SINCE THE BEGINNING of written history we have used the art of ceremony to bring the inordinate to light and to pay respect to important life passages. Over the years we discovered that by weaving a formal service into an event, we were able to bring validity and distinction to our everyday lives, and so we began to expand our use of ceremonies.

We now observe births and birthdays, marriages and anniversaries, graduations and death. There are seasonal sacraments, religious rites, and patriotic performances. Everything from kindergarten graduation to a groundhog seeing his shadow seems to require a certain amount of ceremonial grandeur. And yet there are many important life passages that continue to go unnoticed. Transitions like menarche and menopause are still publicly ignored. Traditionally, the starting and stopping of the menstrual cycle has not been celebrated in western cultures because the menstrual blood itself has been considered a taboo subject; women couldn't celebrate what they couldn't discuss.

Thankfully, times are changing and women not only want to talk about the power of their menstrual blood, they want to celebrate it. These celebrations often take the form of menarcheal and menopausal rites. Like all other truly sacred ceremonies, the menopausal ceremony, which is often referred to as "the crowning of the crone," is a way of publicly acknowledging the completion of a life changing transition. The transition in this case is the menopausal woman's journey to her inner isle and back. And the moment she steps back into the outer world and begins to share her gifts, she leaves behind her years of childbearing and begins her years as bearer of the spirit. She is now a wise-woman or "she-who-holds-the-wise-blood-within."

Although a woman is symbolically crowned a crone the moment she reenters the outer world and begins to share her wisdom with others, the official celebration of her crone years can take place at any time. In many spiritual circles the formal celebration takes place on the fourteenth new moon after a woman's last period. To make it easier to keep track of, some women choose to celebrate it twelve months from their last period. Still others, who may have forgotten exactly when their last period occurred (or for various other reasons), choose to celebrate it on a birthday.

Whenever a woman chooses to acknowledge that she has entered the crone years, the commemoration should be seen as a milestone and a true celebration. For the crone ceremony is a way of publicly showing the wise-woman that she is loved and valued, not in spite of her age but because of it. The crone ceremony is, in essence, a validation of the incredible journey that the woman has taken in order to reach the crone status.

Like all good parties, "The Crowning of the Crone" ceremony needs a lot of participants. These participants, or guests, should be of various ages. In order for the tradition to endure, there must be a younger generation present that will not only witness the ceremony, but be willing to pass it on. That is why it is just as important to have young maidens and child-bearers at the ceremony as it is to have a few crones.

Each guest attending the ceremony should be asked to dress according to their status. Women who are in their childbearing years should wear red, maidens (who have not yet had their first period) are to wear white, and crones should dress in black. White symbolizes the maiden years because it is the color of innocence and purity. Red is used to celebrate the childbearing years because it is the color of blood and of life. Black represents the crone years, not because it is a symbol of death, but because it is a symbol of the mysteries of life that the crone now carries within her. It is also used because it signifies the spiritual pinnacle of the crone years. Each guest should be asked to bring an item found in nature to the party, such as a flower, a leaf, a rock, or a branch from a tree. During the ceremony, the gifts will be placed in a basket for the guest of honor to keep.

The guest of honor should come dressed as the Goddess, for that is who she now symbolizes. Or if she so chooses, she can be dressed in black to symbolize that she has entered her crone years. She should also wear a headdress of flowers or leaves to indicate she has achieved wisdom and power. This headdress can be made beforehand by the hostess, or it can be made at the party with the help of the guests. If flowers are used, they should be exotic, for they symbolize the exotic and unique nature of the Goddess/crone. Perennial flowers such as the iris are perfect for the headdress because they represent vibrance, beauty, and the ability to withstand all types of weather. If leaves are used, they should also be strong and resilient, such as ivy, passion vine, or moon vine. Another good choice for leaves and flowers might be the magnolia. Magnolias are known for their large, white flowers and their evergreen leaves. The other crones present at the party should also wear a wreath of flowers and leaves to celebrate their own wisdom and power.

The ceremony itself should consist of three segments: the storytelling, the declaration, and the initiation. Items that will be needed for the ceremony include red, white, and black candles for the guests; a black candle for the guest of honor; a basket for the items from nature; and a mirror.

The ceremony begins with all the guests sitting in a circle around the guest of honor. The guest of honor is then asked tell at least two stories: one from her maiden years and one from her childbearing years. She may also share her spiritual journey through menopause with the group, or she may share a related tale such as that of the sealskin. Storytelling is an intricate part of the crone ceremony because it symbolizes a wise-woman's ability to bring back the knowledge from her inner island and share it with the world. It is also a healing tool for the other guests at the ceremony, as it prepares the way for their own menopausal journey.

After the stories have been told, the basket is passed around to all the guests in the circle, from left to right. Each guest places her nature gift in the basket and gives an explanation as to why she chose it. These offerings from nature represent the gifts that the crone bestows upon the world when she shares her wisdom. They also symbolize her ties to Mother Earth.

The next segment of the ceremony is the declaration. This is the part of the ceremony where the soon-to-be initiated crone is asked to proclaim her transformation from childbearer to crone. At this time, a mirror is given to the guest of honor. As she studies her own reflection, she is to read a prepared declaration of her status as a crone. An example of the declaration might be the affirmation for "The Crowning of the Crone" that is found in the Affirmation section of this book.

The final segment is the initiation itself. The initiation begins with the hostess circling the group, lighting everyone's candle with the exception of the guest of honor's. A guest who has either been initiated as a crone, or is postmenopausal, lights the guest of honor's candle, pronouncing her officially a crone. If there are no postmenopausal guests present, then the hostess may perform this last rite. After the guest of honor has been pronounced a crone, she is then acknowledged as a wise-woman by all the guests. This acknowledgment can be an informal greeting or it can take a symbolic form—such as each guest saying, "I welcome you as wise-woman and crone." Either way, it should be performed after all the candles have been blown out.

All in all, the ceremony to crown a crone lies in the individual tastes of the guest of honor and the hostess. The ceremony can be further personalized with a birthday cake and candles, religious statements, or spiritual sayings. Prayers can be read individually, or said out loud as a group. The above rituals can be rearranged, added to, or left out all together, for just as each woman moves through the journey of menopause in her own individual manner, each ceremony to celebrate the journey should likewise be unique.

APPENDIX

THE SPIRITUAL DANCE
OF THE FEMALE
REPRODUCTIVE SYSTEM

SINCE THE DISCOVERY of estrogen and progesterone in the early 1900s, much has been said to undermine and negate the importance of these minute chemical messengers in a woman's body. Even in this enlightened age, patriarchal society continues to make degrading jokes about the effects that hormones have on a woman's competency. Men, and even many women, caught up in the testosterone driven outer world, contribute to this demoralization by claiming that there are no real physiological differences between males and females. But the truth is that men and women are very different, and in more ways than the obvious anatomical ones.

The diversity that separates the sexes lies not in the hormones themselves, though, but in the sacred blueprint of God's divine plan for creation.

While men are, themselves, wondrous creations of God, they do not move through the same type of hormonal dance that women do. And although many would say that is a blessing, it is also a misgiving. For it is through this circular dance that women become anointed with the life-giving force of nature. It is through the raging and diminishing hormones and cycles of blood that the feminine spirit creates and prepares to give life, and creates and prepares to give life again and again.

In fact, from menarche to menopause, a woman's body will reenact the 28 day creation ritual over 1,500 times. This ongoing reenactment of divine creation is what ties her to the inner world, and it is what keeps her seeking God's purpose in everything she does. It is also why, I believe, that women have always been, and will continue to be, the keepers of spirituality.

And what does spirituality have to do with hormones and menstrual cycles? A lot. Because the female body was designed to channel the energy of creation, it is, by its very nature, a vessel of divinity. And as a vessel of divinity, it follows the laws of nature and God. Like everything in the universe, from planetary orbits to the healing mandalas discussed in chapter five, a woman's menstrual cycle is circular. It is a continuous sphere of beginnings, peaks, and cessations. It is an example of Mother Earth's ongoing seasons of death and rebirth, and death and rebirth again. And, more importantly, the menstrual cycle it is a reflection of God's ideas illuminating mankind.

Whether the outcome of the creation ritual is successful and a child is brought forth into the world or not, the dance that the female hormones go through in order to prepare for the divine event of giving birth is and of itself, truly a wonder. Erica Jong wrote a poem titled *Ordinary Miracles* about the ordinary yet miraculous process of her daughter's birth. The ordinary yet wondrous process that it takes to generate a child is just one of hundreds of ordinary yet miraculous creation rituals that go on in a woman's body during her childbearing years. When a child is brought forth, the outcome of the ritual is, of course, different. But the fact remains that the remarkable process that it took to create that baby occurs at least 1,499 other times in a woman's life.

These 1,500 or so monthly miracles are just a few of the countless examples of God's desire to express life in a circular, never-ending pattern. The divine, spherical pattern of the menstrual cycle can be found in every form of God's creation—from atoms to astrophysics. The galaxies and the planets themselves are capitulated by the rhythm and pattern of this great, mysterious blueprint. One of the most obvious and easily understood of these patterns can be found in the phases of the moon.

In new age circles, a woman's period is actually referred to as her moon cycle. The relationship between women and the moon is anything but new, though. The speculative correlation between women and their lunar sister has been going on since history has been recorded. In the days of King Arthur it was reported that the priestesses of Avalon painted a half moon on their foreheads to symbolize their loyalty to their Goddess, and an act called "drawing down the moon" was performed at the full moon to increase a woman's spiritual power over her world.

Although she may no longer paint a moon on her forehead, it is a rare woman who does not in some way feel a mystical connection to the moon. To understand a deeper spiritual meaning of why this is, one would need to understand the phases of the moon and its relationship to the earth and the sun. The sun, and the light that it gives, is much like the spiritual illumination of God; it is invigorating, energizing, and empowering. It is what encourages growth and prosperity. The moon, the earth, and the other planets in our solar system are, of course, the recipients of this light. As the earth spins on its axis around the sun, the side that is facing the sun receives direct sunlight. The side of the earth that is not facing the sun receives its light from a reflection off of the moon.

As the moon orbits the earth, it moves through phases in which it reflects the sun's light in varying degrees. In the earliest stages of its rotation, the moon is said to be waxing, which means that is moving in a way that reflects increasing amounts of light. This waxing is a birthing of sorts, a birthing of light, and it is characteristic of the follicular phase—or first 14 days—of a woman's cycle when she is also preparing to give light and life.

During these first two weeks of its rotation cycle, the moon reflects only a partial light. However, as it reaches the 14th day of its cycle it is in position to fully reflect the sun's rays and radiates brightly in the night sky in what is known as the full moon. This full moon can be compared to a woman's cycle when she is ovulating, or giving birth to the fullness of God's light. It is at this time of the full moon that a woman also becomes round and complete and filled with anticipation and excitement as the life force/seed in her breaks free from her ovaries and moves down to the womb. This is when, physically and spiritually, she is most receptive to God's creative light. It is also when she is full of herself and the power bestowed upon her by her creator.

As the moon continues its rotation around the earth, its fullness begins to wane as the amount of light it is reflecting decreases. This reduction of light is also characteristic of the luteal phase, or second half, of a woman's cycle. During the final two weeks of its cycle, the moon reflects less and less light until finally, on the twenty-eighth day of its rotation, it reaches the phase known as the dark of the moon, or the new moon. This is when it reflects no light. Likewise, in the last 14 days of her cycle, if a woman's seed is not fertilized, than the lining of her uterus (and her light) begins to wane. Once the light of creation has completely dissipated, and the woman is in the dark of her moon and menstrual cycle, she sheds the old and begins again. This shedding, which comes in the form of blood, represents the anointment of divine power. The blood also depicts the spiritual cleansing that must take place before a childbearing woman may begin her cycle again.

Two thousand years ago men mistook this cleansing period to mean that a woman was unclean during her menstrual bleeding. But that cannot be farther from the truth. The spiritual cleansing that a woman goes through during the dark of her moon cycle is merely a release of the old so that she can begin again. And it is why a woman is apt to pull in the mists around her during her period. For she instinctively knows that she must rest and prepare to move into the outer world once more.

As a woman rests and regroups and moves back into the outer world, her cycle begins again. And thus, like the moon, she positions herself over and over to act as a conduit for God's creative ideas in human form. And like her lunar counterpart, the childbearing woman then creates a cycle for light and life on the planet.

However, it is important to keep in mind that this channeling of God's creation through the menstrual cycle does not mean that a woman who has had her uterus removed is no longer considered a divine vessel. Nor does it suggest that a woman is out of sync with the Divine if her cycle does not come every 28 days.

By virtue of their gender, all females hold the power of creation in their consciousness and in their solar plexus from the time they are conceived until the time they die. This powerful connection is programmed into every cell of their beings as long as they are alive on the planet, whether they are having menstrual cycles or not. Furthermore, once a woman has moved into her crone years, she no longer needs the continuous cycles of death and rebirth to remind her of her divinity. For the sacred blood is held within on a continuous basis.

This cyclic rising and falling of the hormones in tune with the universe may seem elementary, but the spiritual dance of the hormones is a complicated one. There are many dancers, many steps, and many tunes that must be played out correctly in order for the dance to be successful. And yet, more times than not, the dance goes on again and again with little interruption. Often the perpetual rhythm is played out in a woman's body for decades without much thought or consideration by her at all. In fact, most women don't even bother to find out the names of the different hormones and how they work until the dance comes to a crashing halt.

It is important, though, for every woman to know how her body works, so that not only will she be able to tell early on if there is a problem with her hormones, but so that she may truly appreciate her extraordinary role in God's divine plan.

I strongly recommend that every woman, whether she is going through menopause or not, read up on how her reproductive system works. It is her Goddess-given right as a keeper of the Spirit to be fully conscious of her part in the divine creation of life. There are many credible books available at local bookstores and libraries that will provide accurate information on how the endocrine and reproductive systems work. Below is a short list and explanation of just a few of the major participants in the spiritual reproductive dance of the sex hormones and how they interact with each other.

Hypothalamus—This tiny gland in the limbic area of the brain (which is where emotions are controlled) is the conductor of the hormonal dance. It puts out the *releasing hormones* that, among other things, tell the pituitary gland when to start the dance (or when to stimulate the ovaries and adrenals into producing sex hormones).

Pituitary Gland—This is the co-conductor of the dance. Also located in the limbic area of the brain, it sends out *stimulating hormones* that tell the ovaries and other glands what tune to play (or what hormones to make). The pituitary produces FSH (follicle stimulating hormone) during the first half of the menstrual cycle. FSH goes through the bloodstream to the ovary that will be ovulating that particular month and stimulates it into producing eggs. FSH also stimulates the production of estrogen. During the middle of the cycle the pituitary releases LH (luteinizing hormone) which causes one of the eggs to burst from the ovary. Menopausal symptoms start appearing when FSH, in an effort to stimulate the ovary's production of estrogen, gets either too high or too low. (However, keep in mind that FSH is not always the best indicator of whether menopause has begun. The journey through menopause is often started long before the FSH levels change.)

Ovaries—The creator of life is, of course, God. But God's tools are the ovaries and testicles. For they are the glands that fashion and produce the seeds of life. They are the instruments upon which God plays the tune of Her creation. In looking at the pictures of the ovaries connected to the follicular tubes (the avenue through which the eggs move down into the uterus) one might even think that they looked like the hands of God, stretching down to touch the womb.

Uterus—Also referred to as the womb, the uterus is the sacred vessel of the divine as it exists on earth. It is the muscle that holds and embraces life as it forms and matures within the female body. It is no accident that this inverted pyramid also resembles a chalice. For it is the Grail that carries the wine of divinity for all mankind.

Eggs—These are the very seeds of life. They are the gems, the miracles of birth that God has entrusted to Her daughters. Female babies are born with approximately five million, give or take a million, immature eggs called oocytes. Most of the seeds produce estrogen and then die off, but after a female has reached puberty, once a month one (or two) of them springs forth from the ovary and makes the voyage down the fallopian tube into the womb. The Goddess consciousness is stored in the memory of each of these eggs, and it is through these seeds that She dreams the world.

Estrogen—This is considered the main hormone of the female body, because it is the most abundant of the sex hormones. It is made primarily in the ovaries, and it is also produced from androgens in the fat cells and adrenal glands. Estrogen is the juice of God's spirit that resides in every cell of a woman's body. It is the wine in the amulet that a journeying woman retrieves when she makes the trip to Avalon. It is the moist dew that refreshes her sealskin while she lives in the outer world. There is a widely held belief that all postmenopausal women's bodies are estrogen deficient. But this simply is not true. Because estrogen is also made from androgens, and because the wise-woman knows how to preserve what estrogen she still has left, many journeying women have enough of this elixir stored in their bodies to last them through their postmenopausal years.

Progesterone—This is the hormone that sustains the creative Goddess force in a woman's body. It comes from the word gestate, which means to bring forth. Progesterone is a calming hormone that relaxes and readies the womb to give birth to God's ideas (or children). It is the slow song that begins playing halfway through the woman's menstrual dance. At the end of the dance, if a woman has not conceived, the progesterone levels come to a crashing halt. This drop in progesterone and estrogen brings about the shedding of her uterine lining and menstrual flow. Progesterone is also a precursor to estrogen, which means it can be converted into estrogen if needed.

Testosterone—While found in considerably lower amounts than in men, testosterone is still very important to the structure of a woman's hormonal dance. This hormone is the get up and go that moves a woman through her cycle, and it is the steady beat of the drum that keeps the rhythm of the other hormones in tune. It is also the animus, the little man at the helm, that guides her barge on the way to Avalon.

Cells—These microscopic universes, which could be considered the end users of the hormones, are a wonder in themselves. There are over a trillion cells in the female body, and every single one of them utilizes hormones to heal and maintain itself. Information that keeps the cell healthy and active is transferred when the hormone moves through the cell wall, attaches to its specific receptor site, and binds with the cell's DNA. When hormones are depleted and unavailable, the cells of the female body deteriorate and age. The study of the human cell is one of the fastest growing areas in science. With the production of Dolly the sheep, researchers have proven that they can manipulate a single cell into cloning an entire species. And more importantly, they have proven that each individual cell is a species in its own right.

REPLENISHING LOST HORMONES

When I was pregnant with my first child, I decided that I wanted to go through labor the natural way, which to me meant drug-free. At the time I believed that if I alleviated the pain of labor, I would some-how lessen my childbearing experience. I felt that the numbing of my pain would also desensitize my experience and keep me from truly bonding with my baby. Besides, I thought, women have been going through the childbearing experience for years without the help of drugs. Why shouldn't I?

This line of thinking was completely and utterly erroneous. Twenty eight hours of being aware of every nerve cell in my body did not in any way advance the bonding experience between me and my daughter. In fact, refusing the drugs had the opposite effect. I became so overwhelmed by my pain that I missed watching my daughter being born all together. The second time around I knew better. With my son, I received an epidural as soon as I was offered one, and was much more con-scious of the birthing experience. In comparing the two births, I believe that there is no difference in the amount of bonding that occurred.

The lessons I learned from my childbearing experiences stay with me to this day. I no longer look at the "natural process" as always being the best process. I evaluate each situation or illness, and make an informed decision with my physician as to whether medical intervention is necessary. And although I certainly understand the logic when a woman tells me she wants to move through menopause "the natural way," I know, too, that the decision to use a pill or a patch in no way lessens her strength or spirit. Whether a woman elects to take estrogen on a daily basis or not, she is still going to experience the seven sacred rites. She is still going to have to summon the barge, pull down the mists, make the quest for holiness, etc. The only thing that will change is that the overall journey will be made a little more comfortable. There is no rule that says crones don't take hormone replacement therapy, and there is absolutely no reason why the journeying woman should be ashamed to ask for help.

Likewise, a woman shouldn't feel pressured to start hormone therapy just because she is on the voyage. If she isn't experiencing debilitating symptoms, then doing without drugs or herbs is perfectly acceptable. The decision to start on HRT or herbs should be highly dependent on how a woman feels, not how her physician or mate or best friend feels. Just as there are many women who glide through labor in two short hours with very little pain, there are many women who sail through menopause without so much as a single hot flash. The bottom line is that a woman needs to gather as much information about the wide range of choices that are out there before she makes up her mind one way or the other. She should talk to physicians, friends, and women from support groups, and she should read as many books as she can find.

In researching information, I found that the most informative books were usually the most current ones. The medical community continues to learn a lot about HRT and menopause on an on-going basis, and information can quickly become outdated. Also, I would recommend that the journeying woman stay away from books and/or doctors who claim:

1) That a woman *must* go on HRT to be healthy.

2) That a woman *should not* go on HRT because it *causes* cancer.

3) That menopausal symptoms are psychosomatic.

4) That removing a woman's uterus will keep her from experiencing painful menopausal symptoms.

5) That a woman under 45 (or 40, or 35, or any age) is too young to be menopausal.

6) That hormones, or the lack of them, don't affect a woman's mood.

Most of the above fallacies have been debunked, but there are still many uninformed physicians and outdated books that will try to convince a woman to go against what her natural instincts tell her to be true.

Following is a list of hormones, both those that require a prescription from your physician and those that can be purchased over-the-counter, that are currently being used to help alleviate the symptoms of menopause. If you are a woman who is considering hormone replacement therapy, I recommend that you look over the list and make an informed decision with your physician about a regiment that is right for you. Remember that no regiment is guaranteed to work right away. It sometimes takes months to find the right dosage.

Estrogen

A woman's body produces three types of estrogen—17 beta estradiol, estrone, and estriol. Estradiol (E2) is the estrogen that is made by a woman's ovaries and is the strongest and most active of the three. Estriol (E3) is the estrogen that a woman's body produces during pregnancy. Estrone (E1) is made from estradiol and stored in a woman's fat cells, and is the least or weakest of the three estrogens. Since 17 beta estradiol is the strongest, it is the most common form used in hormone replacement therapy. However, there is a form out that uses doses of all three types of estrogen called Tri-est.

Natural Estrogen—Natural is used to describe many things these days. Yet the only type of estrogen that is natural to a woman's body is the estrogen her body makes. And since it is impossible to store or replenish that, the term natural will be used to describe what is most like a woman's own estrogen. The latest consensus is that the closest estrogen to a woman's own, is plant estrogen. Estratab, which is an estrogen pill made from soy and yams, is considered to be a safe, natural alternative to the higher-dosed synthetic pills previously prescribed by physicians. Natural estrogens also come in patch, pellet, and gel form.

Conjugated Oral Estrogen—The most commonly prescribed form is Premarin. Although I've heard some women who were taking Premarin claim that they were taking a natural form of estrogen, that is not true. Unless, of course, the woman happens to be half-horse. Premarin, which includes an estrogen that is taken from the urine of mares (pregnant horses) in a way that is less than humane, is one of the oldest and most widely tested forms of estrogen. I've heard many women say that they feel quite well on Premarin, but I still think it is cruel to make a horse spend its entire pregnancy inside a stall peeing in a cup so that a woman can feel better.

Synthetic Estrogens—These are chemicals that act like estrogen in the body. The most common ones are Estinyl and Estrovis. This is the type of high dose estrogen that is found in birth control pills.

Progesterone

This is the hormone that is released during the second half of a woman's menstrual cycle. Years ago, women going through menopause were put on estrogen alone. Because the uterus was not shedding properly due to unopposed estrogen, many of these women developed cancer of the uterus. Estrogen replacement therapy had a bad name for a long time because of this. Then, several years later, researchers found that if progestin (a synthetic form of progesterone) was added to the estrogen, the chances for uterine cancer decreased. Because the progestin encourages a complete sloughing of the uterine wall, it is imperative that if a woman still has her uterus, she also take progestin or the more natural form, progesterone.

Natural Progesterone—like natural estrogen, this is derived from plants, mainly the wild yam. The PEPI (postmenopausal estrogen/progesterone intervention) study was conducted to see if natural progesterone had the same positive effects on the uterine lining as the synthetic form of progestin. It was shown that 300 or more milligrams of natural micronized progesterone did indeed protect the lining of the uterus against cancer. You can purchase micronized progesterone from a compounding pharmacy, or your doctor can write you a prescription for Prometrium, a natural form of progesterone extracted from wild yams.

Progestin—a synthetic form of progesterone, such as the commonly prescribed Provera, which can have terrible side effects. It is found in birth control pills and morning after pills. In years past, it was thought that synthetic progestin was the only form of progesterone that could help prevent uterine cancer in women taking hormone replacement therapy. Through the PEPI study, researchers now know that natural progesterone can be just as effective.

Androgens

There are four types of androgens produced by the body: androgenstestosterone, androstenedione, dehydroepiandrosterone (DHEA), and dehydroepiandrosterone. Although considered to be male hormones, androgens have a very significant role in the female body.

Testosterone, for example, is responsible for a woman's libido, muscle strength, activity of oil glands, memory, and her overall feeling of well-being. I have heard many women say that they never quite felt right on their hormone replacement therapy until testosterone was added. This is especially true for women who have had an oophorectomy (the removal of their ovaries). After an oophorectomy, testosterone levels can drop as much as 80%. And even women experiencing natural menopause can have a significant drop in testosterone. That is why it is important that a woman have her testosterone as well as her estrogen and progesterone tested if she is experiencing menopausal symptoms.

Testosterone

Natural testosterone—made from soy by a compounding pharmacy.

Mythel testosterone—a synthetic form of testosterone.

Dehydroepiandrosterone/DHEA

Like testosterone, DHEA is made by the adrenals, the ovaries, and by conversion of body fat. Levels of DHEA in men and women peak at around age 30 and decline thereafter. Low levels of DHEA can be responsible for fatigue, loss of memory, and depression.

Delivery Systems

There are a variety of ways to get hormones into a woman's body. The method a woman uses isn't nearly as important as how she feels while using it. Every woman responds differently, so if a woman's delivery system isn't convenient for her or if after a few months she doesn't seem to feel as well as she expected, she should try another method.

Transdermal—In this method, the hormones are absorbed through the skin by use of gel, cream, or patch. I have been told by several women that they never felt well until they tried the patch. My physician tells me that hormones absorbed trans-dermally provide a much more stable level than hormones taken in pill form. Also, because hormones are absorbed through the skin directly into the blood, they bypass the liver.

Subcutaneous Pellets—One or more small pellets about the size of a saccharin pill are implanted just beneath the skin. Although my physician swears, and I've heard other women rave, that women feel so much better when using this method, it didn't work for me. Two hours after I received my two pellets I was crying hysterically. For some reason my body absorbed the pellets too quickly and my hormone levels went through the roof. Although the hysteria didn't last long, I would never have the pellets implanted again. The upside to this delivery method is that it lasts from three-to-six months, and you don't have to worry about your hormones on a daily or weekly basis.

Pills—Taking a pill is the most common and probably the most convenient, next to the pellet. But again, because it must be processed through the liver, it can have side effects for women with liver problems.

Shots—They are given every two weeks or once a month at a physician's office. However, they tend to have a rebound effect. Some women say they feel really good right after they have the shot, but then their hormones rebound severely in the days before it is time for another one, leaving them feeling worse than before.

Herbs, Vitamins and Over-the-Counter Remedies

There are many herbs, vitamins, and over-the-counter remedies for women who are either not bothered by their menopausal symptoms or who choose not to go on hormone replacement therapy. However, it is important to remember that just because something is classified as natural or herbal, doesn't mean it is good for you. This is especially true with vitamins and over-the-counter medicines. Not only can too much or a wrong combination make a woman's symptoms worse, but they can be fatal. It is important that a woman seek the help of a homeopathic doctor or health care specialist before beginning any regimen, even one that might be considered natural.

Herbs to Discuss with Your Physician

Don quai—referred to as the female ginseng. It is often used to regulate monthly periods.

Ginseng—there are several different kinds; Panax, American, Korean, and Siberian. It has estrogen-like effects on the body. However, it can make you anxious if you take too much.

Black cohosh—this also has estrogen-like effects on the body.

Wild Yam—has a calming, progesterone-like effect that aids in menstrual cramps.

Licorice Root—another estrogen-like herb that is also a good anti-inflammatory.

Ginger—has a calming effect on the stomach and nervous system.

St. Johns Wort—a mood enhancer that acts like stronger drugs such as Prozac, but without many of the harsher side effects.

*Susan Weed has a wonderful book out on herbs titled *Menopausal Years, The Wise Woman Way* that is an excellent source for women who wish to ease their voyage with herbs.

Vitamins

Vitamin supplements used to be an option. But now that research shows that we cannot possibly get the recommended daily allowances of suggested vitamins and minerals, they are becoming a necessity. The dosages of vitamins and what vitamins a woman needs during her postmenopausal years is still under debate. As with herbs, a woman should consult her health practitioner before starting any regimen.

Following are some vitamins that have shown to be helpful:

Calcium—a must for strong bones. I take 1,200 milligrams a day, but check with your doctor to see what the right amount is for you.

Magnesium—lessens anxiety and helps reduce the frequency of migraine headaches.

All the B's (B12, B6, etc.)—in order for the B vitamins to work properly, they need to be taken together. There are several good B-complexes available on the market today.

E—great for reducing hot flashes. I believe a woman needs to take at least 600 milligrams in order to lower the frequency and intensity of flashes, but be sure to consult with your doctor first.

C—good for everything from hot flashes to colds. I take at least 1,000 milligrams a day (again, ask your doctor).

Garlic—another good antioxidant that acts like an antibiotic. Be sure and consult your doctor if you are taking a blood thinner though, as garlic has blood-thinning properties.

Acidophilus—helps ward off yeast infections and keeps the "good" bacteria balanced in the bowels.

COQ10—the up-and-coming antioxidant. I use 100 milligrams a day for my prolapsed mitral valve and heart palpitations. Ask your doctor if you should try it.

SYMPTOMS OF MENOPAUSE

These are just some of the symptoms a woman may experience during her journey:

Hot Flashes
Panic Attacks
Insomnia
Depression (crying)
Anxiety
Fatigue
Formication (crawly or itchy legs)
Headaches (migraines)
Shortness of Breath
Heart Palpitations
Vaginal Dryness
Loss of Sexual Desire
Fuzzy or Clouded Thinking
Pain in the Joints
Unexplained Phobias
Bladder Changes
Yeast Infections
Cramps
Dry Skin
Loss of Hair
Weight Loss or Gain
Allergies (Sinus Infections)
Osteoporosis

AFFIRMATIONS FOR THE SEVEN RITES

Affirmations are a succession of words or thoughts that tweak our memory and validate what we already know to be true. They are little reminders to cheer us on our way when the only thing that seems certain is our own uncertainty. And when we feel lost and all alone, they are the specks of candle-light that brighten our field of vision.

During menopause, you will find that there is much to validate, much uncertainty, and many long, dark roads. In the following pages, you fill find an affirmation for each of the seven sacred rites. I hope they help lighten and enlighten your path. Read them all at once, or read them as you find yourself in that particular phase of your journey.

Because the power of voice helps awaken the memory, try repeating them out loud. It is also empowering and energizing if you read them to yourself in the mirror. If you like, you might even write a few affirmations of your own.

Affirmation for Summoning the Barge

It is with an open heart
and open eyes
that I consciously
and confidently
summon the vessel
that will transport
me back
through that ever winding
ever knowing
ever healing
current of transformation
into the wise-woman years.

I call on my animus
and my angels
to voyage with me
as I fully release
my hold on the outer world,
and prepare for the journey
to my inner world
with joyful expectancy
and love.

Affirmation for Pulling Down the Mists

In order to regenerate
and restore
my feminine wisdom
to its rightful state
I recess into
the sanctuary of mists
cloaking myself in God's
infinite love
and care.

It is here
in this most holy of places
where I am one with my creator
that I find the peace
and the strength
and the order
to prepare for my
impending transformation
into the wise-woman years.

Affirmation for the Great Initiation of Perimenopause

My time of initiation is upon me
and though
my apprehension quickens
I hold steady to the certainty
that my pain
is but a narrow gateway
through which I must pass-
a gateway that generations
of kinswomen
have passed before me
and a gateway that many more
will pass behind me.

For as the moon wanes
and the tides ebb
I know that I too
must follow the cycle of nature.
And so I soothe my anxious moments
and I redirect my depressed spirit
for now is the time
to be gentle with the process
of returning home.

Affirmation for the Quest for Holiness

I have lived too long
with outdated, unwanted, and unproductive
beliefs about my own intrinsic worth.

In order to become both holy and whole
I vow to relinquish and denounce
any and all
malignant, oppressive, or painful
emotions, ideas, and opinions
I have about myself and others.

In my quest for holiness,
I forgive those who have
intentionally or unintentionally
hurt me
and I forgive myself for any pain I have
intentionally or unintentionally
inflicted on others.

I honor myself
as a priestess and a divine
spiritual being
and as such
I let go and let God.

Affirmation for Bathing in the Healing Waters

I open my eyes
to the clear, cleansing water
of Truth
and behold
the Goddess
that is my reflection.

I am no longer
enslaved by
the measurements
and dimensions
of the outer world.

Acceptance is the remedy
for what ails me, now.

I celebrate my roundness
as I am encircled
and made whole
by God's divine
healing presence.

Affirmation for Holding the Blood Within

The moment is here
I have arrived.

The long and painful voyage
that I thought would never end
is over.

The blood and the energy
that have been seeping from my womb
out over the world
for decades
are now held within
and
I feel their power quicken
in my solar plexus
as I stand on the threshold
of Avalon
waiting to take my first
steps as full-fledged
priestess and
wise-woman.

Affirmation for the Crowning of the Crone

I am a woman of old
though not of years
but of wisdom and spirit.
I am full-fledged priestess.
I am a crone.

Within my belly resides
the wise-child
and the wise-woman
of my ancestors.

I am both whole and holy.

I go forth to replant
and reseed my people
with the wisdom I have learned
on my long journey inward.

It is with a light heart
and a strong mind
that I recant the story of my travels
for I am a seeker of Truth
and a daughter of the highest being.

I am a woman who has made it
to the ends of Mother Earth
and back again.

GLOSSARY

Adrenal Glands—Two glands located just above the kidneys that produce hormones and control stress.

Androgens—Although considered to be male hormones, androgens have a very significant role in the female body. They are responsible for a woman's libido, muscle strength, and overall sense of well-being.

Avalon—The island of paradise in Arthurian legend where the Goddess was worshipped. It was where King Arthur was taken when he died. During menopause, it represents the inner isle of a woman's soul.

Barge—The ethereal vessel that symbolizes a woman's ability to transport herself through any crisis.

Crone—At one time it depicted an old and haggard-looking woman. It is currently used to describe a postmenopausal woman who shares her wisdom with the outer world.

Endocrinologist—A physician who treats the endocrine system. He/She often specializes in hormonal imbalances.

Estrogen—A hormone secreted primarily by the ovaries, adrenal glands, testicles, and fat cells. The three major types of estrogen are estradiol, estrone, and estriol. Estradiol is the estrogen that is produced by a woman's ovaries, and is the strongest and most active of the three. Estriol is the estrogen that a woman's body produces during pregnancy. Estrone is made from estradiol and stored in a woman's fat cells, and is the least, or weakest, of the three estrogens.

Excalibur—The legendary sword of King Arthur. During menopause, forgiveness becomes the excalibur, or swift sword, of the journeying woman who wishes to free herself of past experiences.

Follicular Phase—The first half, or first two weeks, of a woman's menstrual cycle. During this stage, the uterus is building up its lining in preparation for the egg that is about to be released from the ovary.

FSH—Follicle Stimulating Hormone. Produced during the first half of the menstrual cycle by the pituitary gland, FSH moves through the bloodstream to the ovary and stimulates it into producing eggs. FSH also stimulates the production of estrogen.

Grail—According to medieval legend, it was the large, round cup that was used by Jesus during the last super. This cup was sought after by King Arthur's knights, and is often used to signify other holy quests.

HRT—Hormone replacement therapy. It refers to the artificial replacement of estrogen and progesterone in a woman's body.

Hypothalamus—A gland in the limbic area of the brain that puts out the releasing hormones that tell the pituitary gland when to stimulate the ovaries into producing sex hormones.

Hysterectomy—The removal of the uterus.

Inner world—An internal existence where the majority of little girls live before puberty, and where the majority of women retreat when they go through menopause. Being in the inner world means being fully present in the inner, spiritual world of one's being.

Initiation—The onset or beginning of a new experience. During the journey of menopause, a woman is initiated into her wise-woman years during the phrase known as perimenopause.

LH—Luteinizing hormone. It is produced mainly by the pituitary gland and is released during the second half of a woman's menstrual cycle. The secretion of this hormone is responsible for the egg bursting from the ovary.

Luteal Phase—The second half, or two weeks, of a woman's menstrual cycle. It is the time, after ovulation, when progesterone is preparing the lining of the uterus. If no egg was fertilized, then the lining will be shed.

Menarche—Typically used to describe a woman's first menstrual cycle. But it also denotes the journey through puberty.

Menopause—Typically used to describe a woman's last menstrual cycle, but it also denotes a woman's journey through the final years of menstruation.

Menses—The menstrual flow or discharge of menstrual blood.

Micronized—The reduction of substances to particles so that they can be metabolized easier.

Outer world—An external existence where women find themselves spending the majority of their childbearing years. Being in the outer world means being an active participant in the comings and goings of the physical world.

Ovaries—The two female reproductive glands that produce eggs and hormones.

Pilgrimage—A spiritual journey.

Perimenopause—The five to ten year period before the cessation of menses. It is often the most difficult time of a woman's journey through menopause

Pituitary Gland— Located in the limbic area of the brain, it sends out the stimulating hormones that tell the ovaries what hormones to produce.

Progesterone—Derived form the word "gestate" which means "to bring forth." It is a hormone that is produced during the second half of the menstrual cycle and it is what prepares the uterus for the fertilized egg. It is also what sustains the lining of the uterus during pregnancy.

Progestin—A synthetic form of progesterone.

Rite—A sacred or ceremonial act.

Soulskin—The sacred covering of a woman's spirit that protects her from harm in the outer world.

Testosterone—A hormone that is made by the ovaries, adrenal glands, and testes. Although found primarily in men, women's bodies also make and depend on testosterone to build muscle.

The Mists—The transparent dividing line between the inner and outer world. They keep the physical and spiritual worlds separate.

Waning—To decrease in size. During the lunar cycle it represents the last quarter when the light of the moon is decreasing. During a woman's menstrual cycle, it represents the luteal phase, or the time after ovulation and before her menses.

Waxing—The molding or making of something. It represents the first half of the lunar cycle when the moon is becoming full. It also represents the first two weeks of a woman's menstrual cycle, or the follicular phase, when her uterus is building up its lining before ovulation.

Wise-woman—A woman who has arrived at the land of her sacred being, had her last period, and then journeyed back to the outer world to share what she has learned with others. At this stage in her life, a woman is said to have accumulated the wisdom of the universe, and holds the "wise blood" within.

BOOK DESCRIPTIONS

The Book of Good Habits
Simple and Creative Ways to Enrich Your Life
by Dirk Mathison
224 pages $9.95

Café Nation
Coffee Folklore, Magick, and Divination
by Sandra Mizumoto Posey
224 pages $9.95

Collecting Sins
A Novel
by Steven Sobel
288 pages $13

Health Care Handbook
*A Consumer's Guide to the American Health
Care System*
by Mark Cromer
256 pages $12.95

Helpful Household Hints
The Ultimate Guide to Housekeeping
by June King
224 pages $12.95

**How To Find Your Family Roots and
Write Your Family History**
by William Latham and Cindy Higgins
288 pages $14.95

**How To Win Lotteries, Sweepstakes,
and Contests in the 21st Century**
by Steve "America's Sweepstakes King"
Ledoux
224 pages $14.95

Letter Writing Made Easy!
*Featuring Sample Letters for Hundreds of
Common Occasions*
by Margaret McCarthy
224 pages $12.95

Letter Writing Made Easy! Volume 2
*Featuring More Sample Letters for Hundreds
of Common Occasions*
by Margaret McCarthy
224 pages $12.95

Nancy Shavick's Tarot Universe
by Nancy Shavick
336 pages $15.95

Offbeat Food
Adventures in an Omnivorous World
by Alan Ridenour
240 pages $19.95

Offbeat Golf
A Swingin' Guide To a Worldwide Obsession
by Bob Loeffelbein
192 pages $17.95

Offbeat Marijuana
*The Life and Times of the World's
Grooviest Plant*
by Saul Rubin
240 pages $19.95

Offbeat Museums
*The Collections and Curators of America's
Most Unusual Museums*
by Saul Rubin
240 pages $19.95

Past Imperfect
*How Tracing Your Family Medical History
Can Save Your Life*
by Carol Daus
240 pages $12.95

Quack!
*Tales of Medical Fraud from the Museum of
Questionable Medical Devices*
by Bob McCoy
240 pages $19.95

The Seven Sacred Rites of Menopause
The Spiritual Journey to the Wise-Woman Years
by Kristi Meisenbach Boylan
144 pages $11.95

Silent Echoes
*Discovering Early Hollywood Through the
Films of Buster Keaton*
by John Bengtson
240 pages $24.95

What's Buggin' You?
Michael Bohdan's Guide to Home Pest Control
by Michael Bohdan
256 pages $12.95

ORDER FORM
1-800-784-9553

	Quantity	Amount
The Book of Good Habits ($9.95)		
Café Nation ($9.95)		
Collecting Sins ($13)		
Health Care Handbook ($12.95)		
Helpful Household Hints ($12.95)		
How to Find Your Family Roots . . . ($14.95)		
How to Win Lotteries, Sweepstakes, and Contests . . . ($14.95)		
Letter Writing Made Easy! ($12.95)		
Letter Writing Made Easy! Volume 2 ($12.95)		
Nancy Shavick's Tarot Universe ($15.95)		
Offbeat Food ($19.95)		
Offbeat Golf ($17.95)		
Offbeat Marijuana ($19.95)		
Offbeat Museums ($19.95)		
Past Imperfect ($12.95)		
Quack! ($19.95)		
The Seven Sacred Rites of Menopause ($11.95)		
Silent Echoes ($24.95)		
What's Buggin' You? ($12.95)		

	Subtotal	
CA residents add 8.25% sales tax		
Shipping and Handling (see left)		
	TOTAL	

Shipping & Handling:
1 book $3.00
Each additional book is $ .50

Name _____

Address _____

City_____ State _____ Zip _____

❏ Visa ❏ MasterCard   Card No.: _____

Exp. Date _____ Signature _____

❏ Enclosed is my check or money order payable to:

Santa Monica Press LLC
P.O. Box 1076
Santa Monica, CA 90406
www.santamonicapress.com

1-800-784-9553